When Love Dies

PERSPECTIVES ON MARRIAGE AND THE FAMILY
Bert N. Adams and David M. Klein, *Editors*

WIFE BATTERING: A SYSTEMS THEORY APPROACH
Jean Giles-Sim

COMMUTER MARRIAGE: A STUDY OF WORK AND FAMILY
Naomi Gerstel and Harriet Gross

HELPING THE ELDERLY: THE COMPLEMENTARY ROLES
OF INFORMAL NETWORKS AND FORMAL SYSTEMS
Eugene Litwak

REMARRIAGE AND STEPPARENTING:
CURRENT RESEARCH AND THEORY
Kay Palsey and Marilyn Ihninger-Tallman (Eds.)

FEMINISM, CHILDREN, AND THE NEW FAMILIES
Sanford M. Dornbusch and Myta F. Strober (Eds.)

DYNAMICS OF FAMILY DEVELOPMENT:
A THEORETICAL PERSPECTIVE
James M. White

PORTRAIT OF DIVORCE:
ADJUSTMENT TO MARITAL BREAKDOWN
Gay C. Kitson with William M. Holmes

WOMEN AND FAMILIES: FEMINIST RECONSTRUCTIONS
Kristine M. Baber and Katherine R. Allen

CHILDREN'S STRESS AND COPING:
A FAMILY PERSPECTIVE
Elaine Shaw Sorensen

WHEN LOVE DIES: THE PROCESS
OF MARITAL DISAFFECTION
Karen Kayser

WHEN LOVE DIES

The Process of Marital Disaffection

KAREN KAYSER

The Guilford Press
New York   London

Library of Congress Cataloging in Publication Data

Kayser, Karen.
   When love dies : the process of marital disaffection / by
Karen Kayser.
      p.   cm.—(Perspectives on marriage and the family)
   Includes bibliographical references and index.
   ISBN 0-89862-086-4
   1. Marriage. 2. Love. I. Title. II. Title: Marital
disaffection. III. Series.
HQ734.K353   1993
306.81—dc20   93-10227
                                                      CIP

To Fred,
who is proof that love
doesn't have to die

Preface

During my experience as a clinician working with couples, I have been fascinated with and challenged by the phenomenon of "falling out of love." A common occurrence in therapy is one of the spouses announcing during the initial session, "I want out." With further questioning, it becomes apparent that the spouse has been apathetic and indifferent about his or her marriage for quite some time and that the current state of desperately "wanting out" did not evolve over night but after months—usually years—of growing dissatisfaction. In fact, these spouses often can tell the therapist exactly when they first had doubts about being married and can relay detailed accounts of significant events or turning points that resulted in the gradual deterioration of love for their partner. I call this process of "falling out of love" *marital disaffection.*

From this experience, I began to ask the following questions: What are these turning points? Does disaffection follow some predictable course or pattern? What emotions, thoughts, and behaviors characterize the process of marital disaffection, and how do they shift during the process? Whereas previous studies have focused primarily on the process of how partners dissolve their relationships, much less is known about how love declines in a marriage that may or may not end in actual relationship dissolution.

This book is based primarily on a research study that involved in-depth interviews with spouses who no longer loved their partner. These spouses recounted stories of how their love diminished over time, starting with first doubts about their marriage to a current state of marital disaffection. Some of the spouses were planning to divorce their partners, while others were committed to "sticking it out"—usually for the sake of their children or because no partner better than their spouse was available.

To understand more fully the factors associated with disaffection, a survey of a large random sample of spouses was conducted. This sample consisted of spouses experiencing varying degrees of marital love and disaffection. Hence, the survey made it possible to compare on several variables spouses who still loved their partner with those who were no longer in love.

Although marital disaffection is a sad and discouraging topic, this book is as much about what makes a marriage successful as what makes one fail. By studying and learning about the dynamics of marriages that produce disaffection, we can better understand what is needed to maintain love in our marriages. Also, recognizing the turning points and phases of this process may alert a spouse or clinician to confront the problems before it is too late.

Plan of the Book

This book will examine the following questions:

- Are there distinct stages of marital disaffection?
- What feelings, thoughts, and behaviors are characteristic of each phase of disaffection?
- Is there a predictable ordering or sequence to the phases of disaffection?
- What are some of the warning signs of a spouse moving toward disaffection?
- How do disaffected spouses differ from nondisaffected spouses?
- What type of help is necessary to restore love in a disaffected marriage?

Chapter 1 looks at how the institution of marriage has been transformed in modern society to one with a growing emphasis on love. The chapter defines the concept of marital disaffection and distinguishes it from other similar concepts, such as marital dissolution, marital dissatisfaction, marital breakdown, and marital instability. Variations of disaffected marriages are examined: (1) disaffected spouses who divorce; (2) disaffected spouses who remain married; (3) couples who recover from disaffection; and (4) unilateral disaffection.

Chapter 2 describes the experience of the disaffected spouses during the beginning phase of marital disaffection when they first had doubts about their marriage. In response to these doubts, the respondents describe how they attempted to change the marriage and how their partner reacted to these attempts. The types of coping strategies used by the respondents to deal with their marital distress are examined.

In Chapter 3 the respondents recount their feelings, thoughts, and actions as they were moving into the middle phase of disaffection. The chapter illustrates the significant shifts in the respondents' experiences from the beginning phase to the middle phase.

Chapter 4 delineates the final phase of reaching disaffection in marriage. It describes the desperate efforts by the respondents to save their marriage and the dilemma of deciding whether to stay or to leave.

In Chapter 5 the reasons for disaffection are explored. This chapter examines the factors reported by the disaffected spouses as causing their disaffection. The factors of mutuality and control, intimacy, attributions, priorities, and alternative attractions are discussed.

Chapter 6 compares disaffected spouses with nondisaffected spouses with findings from a random sample survey of approximately 350 spouses. The relationship of marital disaffection with psychological well-being, commitment, attributions, and gender are examined.

Chapter 7 has a clinical focus. It describes interventions to repair marriages during each stage of the process of disaffection. Interventions are suggested to prevent marital disaffection, address the hurts and anger accumulated during disaffection, facilitate positive interactions, restore feelings of love, and help decision making about the possible ending of a marriage.

Acknowledgments

It has been my good fortune to have worked with Bert Adams and David Klein, editors of the series of which this book is a part. Their suggestions for revision along with their constant enthusiasm for the project have been invaluable. Also, I thank the staff of The Guilford Press and, in particular, Senior Editor Sharon Panulla.

I am indebted to several people for their guidance with the research upon which this book is based. They include Joe Veroff, Oscar Barbarin, John Tropman, and Chris Peterson. Larry Kersten assisted with the early theoretical work on the process of marital disaffection. The University of Michigan provided funding to conduct the research.

My coworkers at the Boston College Graduate School of Social Work and Dean June Gary Hopps have been consistently encouraging. Mary Kelley's typing is much appreciated. Special thanks go to Emily Strainchamps for making the manuscript more readable. I especially want to thank my husband, Fred Groskind, whose patience, encouragement, and understanding during my long work hours are greatly appreciated.

Finally, I am most grateful to the women and men who shared their experiences of marital disaffection with me. Knowing the difficulty of talking about such experiences, I appreciate their willingness to help me in my study of the subject.

Contents

ONE

Love in Contemporary Marriage

1

The Transition to a Love-Centered Marriage 3
The Concept of Marital Disaffection 6
Disaffected Spouses Who Divorce 8
Disaffected Spouses Who Remain Married 10
Couples Recovering from Disaffection 13
Unilateral Disaffection 15
A Process Orientation to Marital Disaffection 17
Overview of the Study 19
Summary 23
Notes 24

TWO

Beginning Disappointments

29

Turning Point Events 30
Disillusionment 32
Attempts to Change the Marriage 35
Reactions of the Nondisaffected Partner 38
Coping Strategies 41
Summary 44
Notes 45

Contents

THREE

Between Disappointment and Disaffection

47

Feelings of Anger   47
Feelings of Hurt   49
Negative Evaluation of Partner   52
Assessing Rewards and Costs of the Marriage   54
Thoughts about Leaving the Partner   57
Continued Efforts to Change the Marriage   60
Physical and Emotional Withdrawal   62
The Partner's Reactions   64
Summary   65

FOUR

Reaching Disaffection

67

Apathy and Indifference   67
Deciding to Dissolve the Marriage   71
Actions to End the Marriage   74
Final Efforts to Save the Marriage   76
The Partner's Reactions to Their Spouse's Disaffection   79
Changes Desired by the Disaffected Spouses   83
Coping with Disaffection   86
Summary   88
Overview of the Marital Disaffection Process   89
Note   90

FIVE

What Causes Love to Die

93

Mutuality and Control   93
Lack of Emotional Intimacy   99
Ineffective Conflict Resolution   101
Shift in Attributions for Problems   104
Individual Happiness Becomes a Higher Priority   112
Alternative Attractions   114
Summary   116

Contents

SIX
A Comparison of Disaffected and Nondisaffected Spouses
119

Marital Disaffection and Psychological Well-Being   120
Commitment and Marital Disaffection   122
Attributions in Marital Relationships   126
Gender and Marital Disaffection   131
Summary   135
Notes   137

SEVEN
Restoring Love in a Disaffected Marriage
139

Early Interventions: Preventing Marital Disaffection   140
Middle Interventions: Reviving the Marriage   147
End Phase Interventions: The Point of No Return?   152
Summary   156
Suggestions for Future Research   157

APPENDIX A
Questionnaire on Marital Relationships
161

APPENDIX B
Interview Schedule
169

References
173

Index
187

Love in Contemporary Marriage

The gods gave man fire so he put it out with water. They gave
him love so he put it out with marriage.
                                                    —SAM LEVENSON (1979)

This joke from the late 1970s stands in sharp contrast to the popular 1950s song that declared that love and marriage are as inseparable as a "horse and carriage" (Cahn & Van Heusen, 1955). It is probably no coincidence that the institution of marriage was most revered during the decade of the 1950s, while a more cynical attitude had emerged by the 1970s. One might go further and say that love, having the strength and vitality of a horse, is what pulls the more static institution of marriage—a carriage—along. If the horse runs off, the unhappy couple is left confined and confused in the box that once seemed to fly them down the road of life.

The institution of marriage by itself is obviously not responsible for people falling out of love. Yet many couples struggle to sustain love in their marriage after the romance of the courtship begins to fade. In fact, it seems much easier to fall into love than to stay in love. The question is, what takes place within some marriages that extinguishes the joy that was felt so powerfully in the beginning? How can feelings of love turn so quickly to apathy and indifference? Although falling out of love does not occur in every marriage, the risk of it has been high enough to make some people reluctant to "tie the knot." Hence, the number of Americans living together outside of marriage has increased tremendously during the last two decades.

Despite the struggles and challenges of maintaining a loving relationship, marriage continues to be popular. While there is a greater tolerance for singleness and nonmarital cohabitation, there still is a strong preference for marriage (Orthner, 1990). Almost 90% of all Americans will marry at least once (Glick, 1989). Even the majority of people who have known the pains of divorce remarry. This means that divorce per se is not necessarily the rejection of the concept of marriage but the rejection of a particular spouse or relationship. In contemporary society, Americans still hold marriage as a more central value than either work or leisure pursuits (Campbell, Converse, & Rodgers, 1976). Other research shows that, compared to the single, separated, divorced, and widowed, married persons generally exhibit better physical health and greater psychological well-being and life satisfaction (Campbell, Converse, & Rodgers, 1976; Gove, Hughes, & Style, 1983; Gove & Shin, 1989; Hafner & Miller, 1991; Ryan & Hughes, 1989; Willits & Crider, 1988).

Clearly, people have high expectations of marriage. When these expectations are not met, disillusion and disenchantment often set in. In fact, a high divorce rate itself may be partly a result of excessively high hopes for marriage, rather than an indication that people are turned off to marriage (Berardo, 1990). With high expectations for finding personal happiness in marriage, individuals may become more easily disillusioned when the partner does not fulfill them. Bardwick (1979) elaborates on this view of marriage and self-fulfillment: "We can predict a higher divorce rate when the criteria of success in marriage change from family integrity, security, and contentment to happiness." (p. 120). Some social scientists view the changing criteria for marriage as a positive sign. The greater emphasis on criteria such as happiness and companionship may mean that those marriages today that stay together are more likely than before to be emotionally rewarding relationships (Popenoe, 1990).

The increased expectations for happiness in marriage have been attributed to the self-fulfillment movement of the 1970s (Bardwick, 1979). But another explanation for the increased pressure on marriage to provide happiness is the growing anonymity and alienation of contemporary society. Lacking close ties with extended family or one's community, people rely totally on their spouses to provide the emotional support and companionship that were at one time provided by a number of people (Kitson, 1992). In short, the *desire* to marry has not changed, but the *expectations* of marriage have.

The Transition to a Love-Centered Marriage

Sociologists Burgess and Locke (1945) were among the first social scientists to write about the dramatic changes in marriage in the 20th century—namely, the transition from the "institutional" to the "companionship" form of marriage. The trend toward a greater emphasis on the fulfillment of love and emotional needs through marriage has been further documented by such researchers as Blood and Wolfe (1960), Veroff, Douvan, and Kulka (1981) and Caplow, Bahr, Chadwick, and Williamson (1982).

The expectation of love in marriage is definitely not new. The concept of romantic love developed during the 19th century when sexuality became tied to both love and marriage. Within the institution of marriage a unique attempt was made to combine romantic feelings with sexuality (Kersten & Kersten, 1988). The idea was conveyed that "love is the ultimate justification for marriage; marriage alone justifies sex; sex and love are therefore the two basic hallmarks of the marital union and neither sex nor love are culturally acceptable outside of marriage" (Crosby, 1985, p. 84). What has changed in the 20th century is the priority and primacy of love in marriage, especially in Western societies.

> It is unlikely that any culture has ever expected as much of the union of one woman with one man as we do in the United States. We are unique, if not in our insistence that we must combine passionate romance with great sex within marriage, then certainly in the naive and intense expectation that romance and sex are and will continue to be the most important in-

gredients in marriage and that little else is really necessary.
(Crosby, 1985, p. 87)

Although love has been historically important in marriage, men and women married and stayed married mainly because of certain legal, social, and economic ties. Choosing a partner was based on whether the husband was a good provider or whether the wife would be a good mother and homemaker. No longer are these considered by most people to be the most important standards for choosing partners.

Even the divorce laws have changed to reflect this emphasis on love in marriage. Traditional divorce laws allowed people to divorce only if there was proof of a spouse's adultery, cruelty, or other wrongdoing. The lack of love was *not* considered an adequate justification for divorce. However, today no-fault divorce laws allow the lack of love to be a sufficient reason to end a marriage.

Given the primacy of love in marriage in our times, it is not surprising, then, that lack of love is the major reason reported for marital breakdown. In recent studies on divorce, separated and divorced individuals indicated that lack of love was one of the top two reasons for marital breakdown, second either to extramarital sex (Albrecht, Bahr, & Goodman, 1983), or communication difficulties (Bloom & Hodges, 1981). In fact, intimacy and love have been identified as the best indicators of whether couples plan to continue or terminate their relationships (Kingsbury & Minda, 1988). These affective variables were more important than factors such as exchange of resources, conflict resolution, and self-disclosure. Thus, as financial, social, and legal obstructions to divorce in the Western world weaken (Trost, 1986), more emphasis is placed on the emotional bond as a motive for staying together.

Is the romantic bliss of a new love strong enough to hold a couple together in a marriage and to survive the travails of married life? Although the maintenance of love and affection is expected by most couples, the divorce rate in the Western world attests to its fragility and vulnerability. Perhaps this is why some scholars on the family call marriage a "weakened" institution and ask what benefits marriage has to offer in the contemporary world (White, 1990). A question that has challenged social scientists, as well as marital therapists, is how does the love and emotional bond that couples claim existed at the beginning of their marriages gradually erode for many of these couples to reach the final point of apathy and emotional estrangement? What happens during the time between the beginning of a marriage full of love, hope, and caring and its end when indifference replaces the feelings that were once present? The breakdown of an emotional bond does not occur abruptly or immediately after the wedding but can occur over months, or more likely years, of more or less continuing dissatisfaction with the relationship. The decline of love does not usually occur as rapidly as the "falling in love" process and, hence, has been described more appropriately as "stumbling out of love" (Douglas & Atwell, 1988).

The startling projection that approximately one half to two thirds of all first marriages formed in recent years in the United States will likely end in divorce (Martin & Bumpass, 1989; Spanier & Thompson, 1984) clearly indicates that the process of marital breakdown warrants our study. Divorce is a major social concern involving emotional pain, grief, financial difficulties, the increased risk of illness, and a sense of personal failure—as well as a costly impact on children. The long-term consequences of divorce for society lead some authors to question the family's ability to fulfill its basic societal functions, namely to rear and socialize children. However, living in an emotionally dead marriage can be just as painful as being physically separated from one's spouse through divorce. In a study of separated, divorced, and married women, married women with poor-quality marriages had just as poor immune functioning as women who were recently separated or divorced (Kiecolt-Glaser, Fisher, Ogrocki, Stout, et al., 1987).

For decades, family sociologists have been studying the causes of separation and divorce (e.g., Glick & Norton, 1971; Goode, 1956, 1961; Kitson & Sussman, 1982; Norton & Glick, 1979; Spanier & Thompson, 1984; Udry, 1966; White, 1990). However, these studies have focused mainly on demographic factors, with little attention being paid to the process of the actual breakup, or to the cognitions, emotions, and behaviors of individuals involved in separation and divorce (Harvey, Wells, & Alvarez, 1978). The focus on demographic variables in divorce research is the result of the common use of secondary data analysis, which often utilizes data collected for other purposes and not to study divorce (Kitson, Babri, & Roach, 1985; White, 1990). Largely ignored in these studies have been the emotional bonds that play a central role in marital relationships and an understanding of the factors that contribute to their demise. However, before we delineate and examine these factors, we need a clearer understanding of the concept of marital disaffection which will be defined in the next section.

The Concept of Marital Disaffection

Marital disaffection is the gradual loss of an emotional attachment, including a decline in caring about the partner, an emotional estrangement, and an increasing sense of apathy and indifference toward one's spouse. By disaffection is meant the replacement of positive affect with neutral affect. In order for disaffection to occur, it is assumed that some positive feelings existed in the beginning of the relationship. This is unlike Cuber and Harroff's (1965) concept of a passive–congenial marriage, in which the spouses never had the spark of love to begin with and were in a sense "nonaffected." The disaffected spouses in my study had the feelings of love and affection, but these feelings died over time. In the disaffected marriage, negative feelings such as hurt and anger begin to predominate, eventually leading to a state of apathy.

Disaffection provides a barometer of the emotional status of the couple. Assessing the level of disaffection is a central task in marital therapy. This information provides clues about spouses' motivation to work on the marriage and the extent to which the marital therapist may be able to help rebuild emotional ties. In this book we will look at what feelings, thoughts, and behaviors occur as a spouse moves through the disaffection process from an emotionally close relationship to a more distant one.

To gain a clearer understanding of marital disaffection, it is important to distinguish it from other similar concepts. These other states may affect or be affected by marital disaffection, but they are not equivalent to marital disaffection. *Marital dissatisfaction* refers to a perceived low degree of adjustment or unhappiness with a relationship (Booth, Johnson, & Edwards, 1983). Certainly the spouse who is experiencing marital disaffection is also likely to be experiencing dissatisfaction. But dissatisfaction can be relatively transitory and can possibly occur simultaneously with some feelings of love and affection. Disaffection is the absence of loving feelings usually occurring after an accumulation of dissatisfactions with the marriage. Similarly, the term *marital breakdown* describes the "decline in the attractiveness of the relationship, turbulence in feelings about the relationship, disturbance in its conduct, and so on" (Duck, 1981, p.1). But it does not necessarily indicate a low degree of love and affection toward the partner.

Marital dissolution involves the ending or permanent dismemberment of a relationship (Duck, 1981) and usually involves the legal act of divorce or permanent separation (Booth et al., 1983). Marital disaffection does not mean the spouses will dissolve their marriage. Many low quality marriages remain intact. However, marital disaffection usually produces *marital instability*, that is, the propensity to dissolve the marriage, even though dissolution may not be the final outcome (Booth et al., 1983). Disaffection is an indicator of the spouse's *feelings* of love and affection for his or her partner; it does not indicate what a spouse will do or how he or she will behave in the marriage. It does not tell us about the interactive qualities of the couple—their style of communication, their methods of problem solving, their level of commitment, and so on. But these are aspects of marriage that are likely to affect or be affected by a spouse's disaffection.

Whereas love and affection are important indicators of marital quality, these constructs are often underrepresented in measures of marital quality. In a review of six of the most popular measures of marital quality (Klein, 1993), only two of the tests included items on affection. None of the tests included items measuring love.

The Marital Satisfaction Inventory (Snyder & Regts, 1982)

provides an exception to the lack of attention to love common in measures of marital quality. This inventory includes a scale on disaffection that measures the lack of love by items indicating lack of affection or understanding from one's spouse, dissatisfaction with the marital relationship, limited common interests or shared leisure activities, and a propensity toward separation or divorce. Clinical and nonclinical populations were compared on Snyder and Regts's (1982) disaffection scale. Disaffection was common in the clinical population but rare in the general population. The authors conclude that for the purposes of discriminating among couples who need clinical intervention, disaffection is a discriminating factor and a critical dimension that is indicative of the potential breakup of the relationship. However, disaffection as measured by these authors appears to be almost the same as marital happiness. Here, it is being defined more narrowly as the loss of affection and lack of an emotional connection in the marriage.

All marriages experiencing disaffection do not look the same or, for that matter, end the same way. There are many variations on the theme of disaffection in the marital relationship. For instance, there are those disaffected spouses who choose to divorce and those who choose to remain married even though the marriage is emotionally vacuous. There are spouses who experience disaffection at one point in their marriage but are able to regain their feelings of love at a later time. In some marriages only one spouse is disaffected but the other continues to remain in love. We will explore these variations on the theme of disaffection in marriage by looking at disaffected spouses who divorce and those who remain married, spouses who recover from disaffection, and marriages in which only one person is disaffected.

Disaffected Spouses Who Divorce

The high divorce rate in American society testifies to the fact that many spouses are unwilling to stay in unhappy marriages. In analyzing the difference between disaffected spouses who "stick it out" and disaffected spouses who leave, the level of commitment in the marriage plays a crucial role. There are several factors that influence a spouse's commitment. One model of commitment emphasizes investment in the relationship as predicting commitment. Investment factors include satisfaction level, investment size, and alternative quality (Rusbult, 1980). Commitment increases with the passage of time when the resources "put into" a relationship outweigh the costs of leaving it (Rusbult, 1980). As the relationship becomes more "valuable"—as the magnitude of the individual's investment becomes larger—commitment should increase. When individuals have little investment in their marriages, spouses are more likely to respond to problems by threatening to leave, separating, or actually divorcing. These spouses feel they have little to lose and what they have is not worth saving.

While internal factors such as rewards and investment in the marriage influence a decision to leave, one cannot ignore external factors when spouses consider the decision to divorce. Drawing upon Levinger's (1976) work, there are two factors that increase the likelihood that a marriage will stay together and one that increases the likelihood it will end. The first factor is the fullness or emptiness of the marriage's *attraction*. *Barriers* to dissolution (e.g., feelings of obligation, moral proscriptions, community stigma, legal and economic constraints, religious beliefs) are another factor. *Alternative attractions* (e.g., the availability of another partner, the desirability of singlehood, means of self-support) are factors that can threaten marital stability. While love (that is, an attraction within the relationship) is an important factor, barriers and alternatives can determine whether the marriage will actually be dissolved.

The barriers to leaving a marriage that influence a divorce decision include: religious beliefs, divorce laws, friends, relatives, neighbors, religious leaders, children, and finances. All these factors, which have very little to do with love, can discourage people from leaving a marriage. But if these barriers do not exist or exert very little influence on the disaffected spouse, the person is much more likely to leave the marriage.

A growing number of spouses are choosing to dissolve their marriages simply because they have some very strong alternative attractions and not because of some overwhelming dissatisfaction with their marriages (Lewis & Spanier, 1979). These alternative attractions are not restricted to relationships but may be a career or a preference for a single life-style. Furthermore, alternative attractions are increasing, especially for women. With more opportunities for women to pursue careers and jobs outside the home, along with their increased earning power, alternatives to a disaffected marriage are more numerous and realistic. Also, as more couples divorce, the pool of alternative partners for spouses in existing marriages increase. The probability increases that some of these available people will appear more attractive than than the current partner. Thus, staying in a marriage will depend increasingly on its intrinsic value, or on "the sweetness of its contents" (Berscheid & Campbell, 1981, p. 222).

Disaffected Spouses Who Remain Married

Despite the weakening of social, cultural, and legal barriers to divorce, some spouses still choose to stay in a loveless marriage. However, the proportion of couples in this category may be decreasing (Lewis & Spanier, 1979). These marriages are referred to as devitalized or conflict-habituated (Cuber & Harroff, 1965), stable–unsatisfactory (Lederer & Jackson, 1968), empty shell (Goode, 1961) or "non-marriages" (Nye & Berardo, 1973). Unlikely to divorce legally, these spouses choose to remain with a partner from whom they are *emotionally* divorced. They learn to tolerate this condition in order to keep the marriage intact.

Recently there has been much interest by researchers in studying the specific factors that may explain these stable unhappy marriage. Commitment appears to be a critical factor in distinguishing spouses who divorce from spouses who choose to remain in a disaffected marriage. But the particular type of commitment of these spouses often is a "social commitment" in which a person's loyalty is based on the perception of moral pressures, other people's views, and societal forces (Johnson, 1982). In contrast, a "personal commitment" is based on the person's liking for the partner or relationship. Hence, with social commitment, it is a sense of obligation to the relationship rather than a positive feeling about the partner that keeps partners together.

Does the type of commitment that spouses make to each other affect their overall level of satisfaction in the marriage? Research studies have shown that a significant decline in personal commitment over the course of a long marriage corresponds with a decline in marital satisfaction (Rollins & Cannon, 1974) and a decline in the expression of love (Swensen, Eskew, & Kohlhepp, 1981; Swensen & Moore, 1979). Swensen and Trahaug (1985), in their research on commitment and long-term marriages, found that those spouses with greater commitment to the partner as a person (compared to those with the lack of commitment to the other as a person) had significantly fewer marital problems and expressed more love to their spouses. In particular, couples who increased their commitment to each other as persons over the course of their marriages had less difficulty in solving the problems between them, setting the goals of their marriage, dealing with their relationships with the other members of their families, and deciding how they would spend their money. Swensen and Trahaug (1985) conclude:

> If the marriage continues, it must be due to some kind of commitment, but what goes on inside of the marriage will be a function of the *kind* of commitment made. If that commitment is to the institution of marriage or the state of being married, then a decline in marriage satisfaction will take place; but if the commitment is to the other person as a person, then the relationship will grow and improve, and the evidence of this improvement will be an increase in the love expressed and a decrease in the problems in the marriage. (p. 944)

Unlike many studies on commitment, these researchers focused on the effect of commitment on the *interpersonal processes* of marriage as opposed to simply the *outcome* such as divorce.

From a large sample of couples ($N = 578$), Heaton and Albrecht (1991) examined the factors that were associated with marriages of low quality for which the risk of separation and divorce was also low. Similar to the previous studies, many of the characteristics of these marriages reflected an ideological commitment to the institution of marriage. Beliefs that marriage is preferable to singlehood, that marriage is a lifetime commitment, and that couples should stay married for the sake of children increased the likelihood of partners' remaining in an unhappy marriage.

Besides commitment, age influences the stability of these unhappy marriages. Aging appears to be a major life-cycle dynamic associated with marital stability (Heaton & Albrecht, 1991). The "investment" of many years in a relationship contributes to its stability. Similarly, another study (Sabatelli & Cecil-Pigo, 1985) found marriage length positively correlated with barriers to divorce for both husbands and wives. This suggests that the longer an individual is married, the stronger the barriers to leaving the relationship. Also, this study found that the more children a couple has the greater the stability of the marriage.

Another significant factor associated with the stable–unhappy marriage involves social contact (Heaton & Albrecht, 1991). Spouses without social contact were more likely to stay in the marriage. This suggests that potential sources of help, receiving help, or spending social and recreational time away from home may be important when individuals are making the divorce decision. In addition, people who believe they have greater control over their lives also seem less likely to remain in an unhappy marriage. Individuals who feel trapped and unable to make changes will stay in an unhappy marriage. Those who think their lives would be worse if they separated also are disinclined to leave.

Rusbult (1980) also examined stable–unhappy relationships—relationships she characterized by "neglect." Neglect is an ineffectual response adopted by a spouse who does not know what to do about a troubled relationship and is not motivated to do much of anything about it. The reaction to relationship problems is to passively let the relationship take its course hoping it will either improve or die. Hence, this inertia results in a devitalized, empty shell type of relationship. Older persons are more likely than younger persons to respond to problems passively with neglect (Rusbult,

1980). An explanation for this age difference is that "older persons in long-standing marriages may simply have fewer stressors in their relationship or may have learned over years of involvement to respond to dissatisfaction more quietly; younger, single persons in relationships of briefer duration may have more serious problems to confront and believe that it is more appropriate to confront them head-on with voice or exit" (Rusbult, 1980, p. 223). In marriages characterized by neglect, it is likely that a low level of satisfaction was experienced prior to the devitalized relationship. A neglect response to relationship problems is more probable among males, older persons married for some time, and spouses with low self-esteem.

In sum, to look only at the emotional fullness (or emptiness) of a marriage gives an incomplete picture of what keeps spouses together. Even if a spouse's love for a partner is minimal, when assessing alternative relationships, or the costs involved in leaving (e.g., shame, guilt, hurt to children), or the other rewards in the relationship (e.g., property, friends, material possessions), the person may decide to stay in a loveless marriage.

Couples Recovering from Disaffection

Marriages with disaffected spouses do not always lead down the path of dissolution, nor do they always end in stable–unhappy coexistence. Some couples pull themselves out of the depths of disaffection and regain the love once lost. Unfortunately, the research on couples recovering from disaffection is quite sparse. The marital therapy literature provides some understanding of what type of therapeutic intervention helps couples to regain love, but we know little about couples who stop the process of disaffection and restore their feelings of love without therapeutic intervention.

The longitudinal research on marital interaction conducted by Gottman and Krokoff (1989) sheds some light on what distinguishes a marriage that can survive conflict and become more satisfying over time from a marriage that succumbs to conflict and becomes less satisfactory. These researchers discovered that behaviors that serve to "keep the peace" in the present may leave conflicts unresolved and may actually undermine the relationship over time (Gottman & Krokoff, 1989). In particular, conflict that is handled with defensiveness, stubbornness, and withdrawal (particularly on the part of the husband), may be harmful to the relationship over time. Conflict-avoiding couples are at some risk for continuing negative feelings and, ultimately, disaffection. Couples who have developed a sense of "relational efficacy" (Notarius & Vanzetti, 1983), that is, the confidence that they can weather conflict together, are more likely to be able to reverse negative feelings that begin to arise.

Some interesting differences in marital satisfaction between spouses have emerged from this research (Gottman & Krokoff, 1989). Wives who are positive and compliant experience less negative affect from their husbands and report high marital satisfaction. But the marital satisfaction of these couples deteriorates over time, largely due to the husband's stubbornness and withdrawal. The marital satisfaction of wives improves over time if wives express anger and contempt during conflict discussions but declines if the wives express sadness or fear. The results suggest that wives should confront disagreement express anger and contempt, and not be overly compliant, fearful, and sad. Husbands should also confront conflict but should not be stubborn or withdrawn. Neither spouse should be defensive.

Similarly, in Rusbult's (1987) research, those partners who chose to respond more directly and actively to problems were more likely to regain their love. Actions such as discussing problems, compromising, seeking help from a professional, suggesting solutions to problems, asking the partner what is bothering him or her, and trying to change oneself or the partner are attempts to rescue something of value that is in danger of being lost. She found that those individuals with good alternatives (e.g., alternative relationship, spending time with friends or relatives, or solitude) were often motivated to take risks in confronting problems in the relationship. These alternatives gave the spouse a source of power for effecting changes in the relationship (Rusbult, 1987). Direct and active responses were more likely among females, individuals with high prior satisfaction with the relationship, and individuals who invested heavily in the relationship.

In addition to skills in handling conflict, often couples must deal with the anger and bitterness that have built up over the years, feelings that have extinguished the love between the partners. Marital therapists recognize the importance of resolving anger and bitterness before a couple can rekindle their love. To deal with accumulated anger and bitterness in the relationship, Guerin, Fay, Burden, and Kautto (1987) have developed a "bitterness protocol," which is an intensive approach to reducing bitterness in the marriage (see Chapter 7).

Unilateral Disaffection

Disaffection is often an internal or intrapsychic process that can be occurring within one spouse and not the other. Even when both spouses are feeling some disaffection, it is likely that they are not at the same level of disaffection. Furthermore, the spouse who is not experiencing disaffection may be "cooperatively or collusively" involved in the development of disaffection (Napier, 1988).

The unilateral nature of disaffection is similar to the one-sidedness of the uncoupling process as described by Vaughan (1986). In the process of uncoupling, Vaughan found:

> Most often, one person wants out while the other person wants the relationship to continue. Although both partners must go through all the same stages of the transition in order to uncouple, the transition begins and ends at different times for each. By the time the still-loving partner realizes the relationship is in serious trouble, the other person is already gone in a number of ways. The rejected partner then embarks on a transition that the other person began long before. (p. 6)

Similarly, spouses may be at very different stages of the emotional uncoupling that occurs in disaffection.

The unilateral characteristic of uncoupling—and similarly disaffection—is especially evident during the first phase, as the dis-affected spouse spends hours quietly ruminating about his or her unhappiness with their partner. Vaughan (1986) describes the si-lent, unilateral process of the first phase with the following:

> We walk around harboring and mulling over the secrets of our unhappiness. Perhaps they are unarticulated in the beginning because our feelings are nebulous. Perhaps they remain un-spoken because we are uncertain as to their cause, their depth, and their implications. Perhaps we are afraid to share them for fear of discovering or validating the other person's unhappiness. For whatever reason, we won't do it until we are absolutely sure. So the dissatisfied partner creates a private niche in which to weigh the fragile, disturbing new notions, to assess present actions and future possibilities, to make estimates, to consider, to reject, to act, to wait, and, perhaps ultimately, to choose. (p. 13)

Without the partner's awareness or input, much evaluation, reflec-tion, and decision making about the relationship are already taking place.

Marital therapists are quite familiar with this unilateral pro-cess. Working with two spouses who are at quite different points in the disaffection process challenges clinicians. In his book *When One Wants Out and the Other Doesn't*, Crosby (1989) describes re-building these marriages as "almost a hopeless task." Written spec-ifically about therapy with these so-called "polarized" couples, Crosby's book offers clinical suggestions for working with these couples from 16 experts in the field of marital therapy. Regardless of the theoretical approach, these experts emphasize the impor-tance of a careful assessment of the intentions of the spouse who declares "I want out" or "I don't love you anymore." Some spouses don't really want out, they may just be threatening their spouse, or expressing years of pent-up anger, or feeling helplessly at an im-passe, or wanting to be taken seriously. Hence, understanding the concept and process of marital disaffection should aid the clinician in deciphering the feelings and desires of the spouse making these statements.

In distinguishing the various types of disaffected marriages, it is apparent that this classification is not static and immutable. A close relationship is a process—couples may move in and out of love; they can become more in love over time; or they may experience a gradual falling out of love over time. One spouse can move in a different direction and at a different pace than the other spouse. Therefore, it is important to examine disaffection as a process. A major purpose of this book is to describe and understand this process of love dying in marriage.

A Process Orientation to Marital Disaffection

A predominant error in most relationship research has been to view relationships as "timeless states or rootless events, rather than a continuous process with temporal energy, changing form, and a place in the history of the participants' lives" (Duck & Sants, 1983, p. 32). Very few studies on marital adjustment and satisfaction take a longitudinal perspective. One exception is a three-wave survey begun by Burgess and Wallin in 1939. Couples were interviewed during their engagement, after being married for several years, and approximately ten years later. Pineo (1961) analyzed the data of the couples at the second wave of interviewing and discovered a process of disenchantment that occurred between the early and middle years of marriage. This disenchantment was evidenced by a drop in marital satisfaction and adjustment, a loss of intimacy, and decreased sharing of interests and activities. Pineo concluded that there is a short-term disenchantment that occurs early in the marriage that is a consequence of the idealization of the partner and intense romanticism during the courtship. In contrast, the disenchantment occurring later in the marriage is the result of unforeseen changes in the couple's situation or in one or both of the partners' personality and behavior.

Dizard (1968) analyzed the data collected during the third wave of the study. He found that the predominant change between the middle and later years of marriage was an "emotional deadening" of the husband–wife relationship. The spouses reported a decline in happiness and love for one another. He concluded that more couples were moving toward than away from an "empty shell" marriage. These changes seemed to be the result of what the husband and wife did after the marriage and could not be predicted by the spouses' relationship during the engagement period or their early marriage. Dizard attributed the emotional deadening to a greater role differentiation in the couple's relationship. He observed that in the early years of the marriage, authority had been evenly distributed, but by the middle years authority was centered around one spouse, or *both* husband and wife took on increasing dominance. As a consequence, there was more frequent and severe conflict in the relationship. Taking a sociological perspective, Dizard related these changes in the couple's relationship to the external world and the occupational demands of the husband in the society. He found little evidence for internal pressures (e.g., birth of a child) causing the changes in the marital relationship.

More recently there has been research on the breakdown of relationships that by looking at the temporal ordering of events has conceptualized breakdown as a continuous process over time. These studies have revealed many different pathways to dissolution, which vary in terms of length of time and sequences (Baxter, 1984; Hagestad & Smyer, 1982; Lee, 1984; Ponzetti & Cate, 1986; Vaughan, 1986). The most common path described by these researchers is dissatisfaction experienced primarily by one partner, the absence of discussion of problems, the lack of adequate conflict resolution, followed by relationship termination. R. Miller (1982) found that the most common sequence to marital breakup involved a decline in feelings of attraction toward the partner, followed by a focus on the barriers to ending the marriage, and finally attention on the attractiveness of alternatives.

My study of the marital disaffection process differs from earlier research on relationship breakdown in several respects. First, of primary interest in this study was the process of marital disaffection that may *or may not* lead to actual relationship dissolution. Previous research has focused only on those relationships that have terminated and has ignored relationships in which the partners are physically together but emotionally apart.

Second, the subjects who were interviewed for my study were all highly disaffected from their partners in comparison to subjects of previous studies. Previous studies did not differentiate subjects on marital disaffection. However, the process of marital breakdown is likely to be quite different for those individuals who are still in love versus those persons who are not in love with their mates.

Third, all of those subjects in the present study who were dissolving their marriages were interviewed before they had legally terminated their marriages. In some of the studies on marital breakdown (e.g., Hagestad & Smyer, 1982; Ponzetti & Cate, 1986) individuals were interviewed at least a year after the divorce. In Hagestad and Smyer's study, a third of the men had remarried at the time of the interview. In Ponzetti and Cate's study, the subjects had been legally divorced for an average of 32.9 months. By interviewing people who are currently married, it was hoped that less distortion may occur during recall and that there would be less motivation to produce a socially desirable accounting of the ending.

Overview of the Study

To begin my study of the process of marital disaffection, I developed a theoretical model of this process.[1] Table 1.1 presents the model, which includes feelings, thoughts, and behaviors that are hypothesized to occur as a person experiences marital disaffection. In developing this model, I relied on my clinical experience and drew from the theoretical work on relationship disengagement of Duck (1982). His model offered a conceptual framework for the phases of relationship breakdown and described three phases that occur before partners dissolve a relationship—intrapsychic phase, dyadic phase, and social phase.

To test empirically this hypothesized model, I first constructed a questionnaire to measure the level of overall marital disaffection (see Appendix A, Part I).[2] I then interviewed 50 highly disaffected

TABLE 1.1 Theoretical Model of the Process of Marital Disaffection

Phase I: Dissillusionment

Feelings: Disappointment, disenchantment with marriage

Thoughts: Awareness that relationship is not going as well as expected; doubts about the partner and about the decision to marry him or her

Behaviors: Attempts are made to change oneself; tries harder to please partner; tries to love harder or to be more attractive

Phase II: Hurt

Feelings: Feeling treated unfairly and abused; lonely

Thoughts: Partner does not understand you; a mental balance sheet of rewards and costs of relationship is kept; awareness that your emotional and social needs are not being met; thinking that you are not important in partner's life

Behaviors: Dissatisfactions about partner and/or the marriage are expressed to confidants; individual attempts are made to try to change relationship or partner's behavior; some reinforcement from others

Phase III: Anger

Feelings: Resentment, hostility, indignation, bitterness

Thoughts: Awareness of accumulation of hurts over time; thoughts center more on partner's behavior and blame is directed toward the partner; negative thoughts about partner begin to outweigh positive thoughts; less trust of partner's actions and motives

Behaviors: Expressing of affect: hurt, anger, disappointment, disgust; confronting partner with grievances; avoiding partner to protect oneself from further hurt; sexual behavior may stop, diminish, or become a "duty"

(cont.)

TABLE 1.1 (cont.)

Phase IV: Ambivalence

Feelings: Alternating between despair and hope about partner and marriage, indecisive, unresolved

Thoughts: Both thoughts about "making marriage work" along with thoughts of giving up; serious evaluation of what it would take to make marriage work compared to giving up; evaluation of alternatives to current marriage; awareness of external forces to stay in marriage (e.g., finances, children, religion)

Behaviors: Initiate counseling or seek informal types of help to assist in sorting out feelings about the marriage; confide in friends and family about problems; look at others as possible partners

Phase V: Disaffection

Feelings: Indifferent toward partner, detached, alienated, apathetic

Thoughts: Little desire to be emotionally close to partner; think partner cannot satisfy your needs; think any changes partner makes are too late

Behaviors: Try to avoid contact with partner as much as possible; no desire for physical touching of any kind; only "small talk" in marriage; pursue other interests and relationships outside of marriage

spouses using a semistructured interview schedule (see Appendix B). The interview was intended to chart changes over time in marital disaffection. Questions were posed regarding major turning points in their marriages, points at which the disaffected spouses had doubts about their partner and their marriage. The events were not necessarily major catastrophes but were perhaps crystallizing events after a cumulation of a number of things: "the straw that broke the camel's back." In this respect, marital disaffection may be viewed as a chronic, nagging stressor, as in McCubbin and Patterson's (1982) stress model. Events pile up during the marriage until their accumulation leads to a high level of disaffection. So it is not the turning points per se but the "pile up" effect of these points that lead to the high level of disaffection. For each turning point identified, I asked about the respondent's feelings, thoughts, and behaviors at the time. I was interested in finding out to what degree these feelings, thoughts, and behaviors shifted during the process.

To recruit disaffected spouses, notices regarding the study were placed in local newspapers and on bulletin boards of therapists' offices in group practices in a metropolitan area. The notices requested respondents who were experiencing marital difficulties or who were recently separated. To select disaffected individuals, potential respondents who responded to the ad were asked to answer "yes" or "no" to five statements regarding their degree of love and affection for their partner, their desire to confide in their spouse, their ability to forget past hurts in their marriage, the degree to which their love for their partner had increased, and their desire to spend time with their partner. These items were taken from the marital disaffection questionnaire and had the highest correlations with the total score of the disaffection scale. Individuals who answered at least four out of the five questions in the direction of marital disaffection and who were still legally married were invited to participate in the study.

At the time when the 50 spouses were interviewed, they were given the entire disaffection scale. The possible range of scores on the disaffection scale was 21 to 84; the mean for the respondents for this study was 70.8. Compared with a mean of 33.7 from a previous random sample of spouses from the general population (Kersten, 1988), these respondents showed a high level of disaffection.[3] The interview data from one respondent who had a score of 36 on the disaffection scale was omitted from the data analysis.

Of the remaining 49 spouses, 35 (71%) were females and 14 (29%) were males. The respondents' ages ranged from 21 to 68, with a mean age of 37. None of the respondents were married to each other. The length of marriage ranged from 2 years to 39 years, with a mean length of 13 years. About 16% of the respondents had been previously married, and approximately 78% had children resulting from their current marriage. Among the categories for income and education, the average yearly household income was $40,000 to $49,999; average education level was "college graduate."[4] The respondents for this study were married at the time of the interviews, though some had filed for divorce or were contemplating it. A few respondents were separated. Still others were committed to staying in their marriages even though they were highly disaffected.

The length of the process of disaffection of the 49 respondents varied from 1 to 38 years, with an average of 11 years. Each respondent's disaffection process—regardless of its length—was divided into fifths to correspond with the five phases of the hypothetical model. Each turning point event, along with its accompanying feelings, thoughts, and behaviors, were placed into one of these time periods. Upon studying the data from the interviews, I found that instead of five distinct phases, only three phases emerged—beginning, middle, and end.[5]

Summary

Most people expect to have a love-centered marriage. However, many spouses struggle to sustain the love that was experienced in the beginning of marriage. The gradual deterioration of love and loss of an emotional attachment is referred to as marital disaffection.

Marital disaffection is a process that is marked by phases and turning points in a person's marriage. While disaffection may influence or be influenced by other aspects of marital quality (commitment, satisfaction, happiness, stability), it is not the same thing as these other aspects. The concept of disaffection reflects specifically the emotional state of the marriage—the feelings of love, caring, and affection toward one's spouse—and not the actual behaviors of the spouses. This emotional aspect of marriage has been underrepresented in previous studies examining marital quality, even though love is the primary reason many individuals marry and remain married.

Marriages experiencing disaffection are not all the same. For some couples, marital disaffection will result in divorce. However, some disaffected spouses choose to remain married even though they no longer love their partner. Factors such as commitment, barriers to divorce, alternative attractions, and age can impact one's decision to dissolve the marriage. Some spouses are able to regain their feelings of love after experiencing a period of marital disaffection. These couples usually have acquired good conflict resolution skills and are able to deal with anger and bitterness that have accumulated over time.

Spouses in the same marriage may differ on their level of marital disaffection. In some cases, both spouses may be experiencing disaffection, whereas in other cases of unilateral disaffection only one spouse is disaffected while the other continues to love their partner. In the cases of unilateral disaffection, much decision making about the relationship may be taking place by the disaffected spouse without the partner even being aware of it.

To begin the study of the process of marital disaffection, a theoretical model of five phases was developed. Then highly disaffected spouses were interviewed regarding the course of their disaffection. Based on their accounts of this process, the hypothetical model was revised to include three distinct phases. The following chapters describe these phases.

Notes

1. A description of this study and the results appeared in Kayser (1990). Copyright 1990 by The National Council on Family Relations. Adapted by permission. Portions of Chapters 2 to 4 also appeard in this article.

2. The questionnaire contained a Likert-type scale of disaffection (see Appendix A, Part I). The disaffection scale included items from Rubin's (1973) love scale and items from Schaefer and Olson's (1981) Personal

Assessment of Intimacy of Relationships. The remaining questions were originally developed.

In developing the marital disaffection scale, I administered an initial 27-item version of the scale to a nonrandom sample of 76 spouses. This version of the scale correlated highly ($r = .93$) with another scale of disaffection (Snyder & Regts, 1982). In addition, it correlated inversely with general questions on marital happiness ($r = -.56$) and marital closeness ($r = -.61$). On the basis of these correlations, six items were eliminated from the initial version to yield the final 21-item version used in these analyses. The Cronbach's coefficient alpha obtained for the internal reliability of the disaffection scale was .97.

A factor analysis was performed on the disaffection scale by using a principal components analysis with an alpha extraction and varimax rotations. A random sample of 354 spouses (who were not married to each other) was used. Table 1.2 contains the factor loadings for three factors that

TABLE 1.2 Factor Loadings for 21 Measures of Marital Disaffection ($N = 354$)

Measure	Attachment	Emotional estrangement	Emotional support
Look forward to seeing spouse	.72	.33	.00
Miserable without spouse	.67	.00	.00
Enjoy being with spouse	.65	.31	.33
Miss my spouse	.63	.00	.00
Love has increased	.61	.42	.37
Feel close to spouse	.59	.37	.46
Enjoy time with spouse	.58	.00	.00
Enjoy sharing feelings	.52	.00	.50
More positive thoughts	.47	.00	.42
Withdrawing more and more	.33	.66	.45
Apathy and indifference	.00	.66	.00
Avoid spending time	.39	.63	.00
Little desire for sex with spouse	.35	.59	.00
Unconcerned with marital obligation	.00	.52	.00
Spend less time with spouse	.50	.51	.33
Do not feel great deal of love	.33	.42	.39
Turn to spouse with problem	.44	.00	.66
Spouse is always there	.00	.00	.58
Difficult confiding in spouse	.00	.35	.58
Feel lonely with spouse	.00	.44	.55
Angry feelings toward spouse	.00	.47	.52

emerged from the analysis. Because these factors are not distinct, the scale appears to be unidimensional.

3. Some studies would lead us to believe that disaffection in marriage is rampant—at least among women. In her study of 4,500 women Hite (1987) found that women of all ages increasingly express emotional frustration and gradual disillusionment with their personal relationships with men over time. An overwhelming majority of her respondents desired basic changes in their personal relationships with men (98%), stated that they were lonely in these relationships (82%), reported painful and condescending attitudes on the part of their male partners (79%), fought for their rights and respect (78%), and stated that men often seemed not to really hear them (84%). However, Hite's sample emerged from an extremely low response rate (4.5%), which raises serious questions regarding the generalization of her findings to the larger population. A dismal perspective of love relationships is also found in many self-help books—especially those written for women—and these books often espouse the inadequacy of men in close relationships. Many of the popular self-help books are not based on empirical data.

Other studies of marital happiness present a quite different picture. Veroff, Douvan, and Kulka's (1981) national survey found 80% of the respondents rating their marriages either above average or very happy. Another national survey (Campbell, Converse, & Rodgers, 1976) found 90% of the respondents rating their marital satisfaction from above average to high.

To determine more about the frequency of disaffection in marriage, the questionnaire on marital disaffection which was used with the interview respondents had previously been sent to a random sample of spouses in a metropolitan area in the Midwest. Three hundred and fifty-four people responded to the survey (54% return rate)—59% were females and 41% were males. Their ages ranged from 21 to 84, years and they were married from 1 year to 58 years. Eight percent of the sample scored "high" on marital disaffection and another 12% scored "above average." Thus, 20% of the sample were experiencing at least some degree of marital disaffection. This is a small percentage compared to what Hite described in her 1987 study. However, I did find that women were more likely than men to score high on disaffection.

4. The average joint income of the interview subjects ($40,000–$49,000) was close to the estimated average household income of $40,910 for 1988 for the metropolitan area from which the sample was derived (*Editor and Publisher Market Guide*, 1988). The interview subjects tended to be highly educated in that 51% of

the sample were college graduates compared to 40% of the total population (25 years or over) of the metropolitan area (U.S. Bureau of the Census, 1980). The percentage of college graduates could be somewhat higher now since the 1980 Bureau of the Census statistic is outdated, but it is also likely that college graduates may be more prone to respond to a research ad than those without a college degree.

5. The interviews were audiotaped and transcribed. To develop the coding manual used in the content analysis, all the responses to the questions were placed in categories for each variable (e.g. turning point, feeling, thought, behavior, attribution, coping strategy) until all of the responses were categorized. The interviews were coded by two university students who were trained in the coding system and by the author. The intercoder agreement for the interviews ranged from 78% to 96% agreement. Hence, the coding system's reliability was adequate.

Frequencies for each variable in the phases—feeling, thought, behavior, attribution, and coping strategy—were calculated. The sign test was used to compute the degree of change in these variables from one phase to another. This nonparametric test of significance determines the probability of change between pairs of observations of the same individual (Wright, 1976). The SPSS-X statistical package was used in the computation of this test.

T·W·O

Beginning Disappointments

He wasn't intimate. He was before I married him. He really was, and that is something I need—I need to have someone that I can share time with—all of me—my thoughts, feelings, everything. He just stopped doing that, and the whole marriage got mechanical. And just the communication—there wasn't any— everything was taken for granted with him. This is the way we do it, and there's no need to talk about it. . . . He was like that before we were married, but if I complained about it, he was quicker to change it because he did want to marry me, and he didn't want to lose me. But after we were married, it was like "Well, I've got her now, I don't have to change."

(31-year-old female, married 3 years)

The ink is barely dry on the marriage license when doubts and disillusionment about marriage and the partner can begin to set in. For some respondents the doubts started on their wedding day or during their honeymoon. For example, one man, married 2 years, had doubts during the wedding ceremony when he bent over to kiss his bride and she turned her cheek. Shocked by her response, he thought, "What have I done? This was supposed to be the beginning?" When asked how he handled the situation, he responded, "I guess I pretty much shrugged it off at the time. But still there was some underlying resentment."

When asked about their first doubts about their marriage, approximately 40% of my sample identified marital doubts occurring during the first 6 months of their marriage. Another 20% experienced doubts between 6 months and 1 year. Thus, more than half (60%) of the respondents were experiencing dissatisfactions and serious doubts about their marriages during the first year. For the remaining 40% of the respondents, disaffection started to set in later in their marriage.

Turning Point Events

To identify the phases of disaffection, I asked the respondents about turning points in their marriage when they began to have serious doubts about their partner and questioned their love for their spouse. Asking the respondents to identify specific turning point events helped them recall significant feelings, thoughts, and behaviors during the disaffection process. For some of the respondents, the disaffection process had started many years prior to the interview. Therefore, eliciting a specific turning point event from these respondents, as opposed to asking them to give the story of their marriage, made it much easier for them to recall an experience that had occurred a long time ago. This method facilitated recall, a common problem when using a retrospective design.

All the turning point events that were identified during the whole process of disaffection were put into 20 categories which are listed in Table 2.1. The most frequently cited types of events were: partner's controlling behavior (53%), partner's lack of responsibility (49%), and partner's lack of emotional support (47%). A common example of the partner's controlling behavior was unilateral decision making by the partner, which disregarded the respondent's opinion. These decisions often included how the respondent should dress, where they should live, how they should spend money, and so on. Some of them appeared to be major life decisions, others appeared quite minor. But the common element was the lack of consideration for the respondent's input, opinions, and feelings in making the decisions.

The second most frequent type of turning point event, partner's lack of responsibility, was characterized by breaks of trust, unequal sharing of family responsibilities, and other irresponsible

TABLE 2.1 Turning Point Events during the Marital Disaffection Process

Events	Percent[a]
1. Partner's controlling behavior	53
2. Partner's lack of responsibility	49
3. Partner's lack of emotional support	47
4. Partner's substance abuse	29
5. Other undesirable trait of partner	27
6. Partner's relationship with children	27
7. Stressful event	20
8. Partner's verbal abuse	20
9. Respondent's personality changed	18
10. Respondent's awareness of incompatabilities	18
11. Partner's extramarital affair	18
12. Partner's lack of self-disclosure	16
13. Partner's physical violence	14
14. Partner's sexual problems	14
15. Respondent's extramarital affair	10
16. Interference of in-laws	10
17. Physical separation	10
18. Respondent's depression	8
19. Negative evaluation of marraige by outsiders	8
20. Discussion of separation with partner	4

[a]Percentage of respondents ($N = 49$) who cited the event as a turning point in their marriage; total is more than 100% because of multiple responses.

acts. Examples included going to jail for drunk driving, leaving children unattended, losing jobs, spending inordinate amounts of time with friends, and so on.

Events that were categorized as partner's lack of emotional support involved a lack of care and concern for the respondent, usually during a stressful event such as a pregnancy, birth of child, or death of a family member.

Regardless of when the first phase of disaffection began or how long it lasted, the accounts of the first phase contained some common characteristics. What follows is a description of the first phase of disaffection as reported by the respondents.

Disillusionment

During the beginning of the process of marital disaffection, most respondents experienced feelings of anger and hurt. In fact, these two emotions were ubiquitous throughout the whole process of disaffection. However, unique to the beginning phase was the feeling of *disillusionment*. Spouses stated that they were disillusioned with their partner[1]; that is, the partner's behavior was not what they had expected. The reality of their marriage and their partner was not living up to their dreams, fantasies, and expectations prior to their marriage. This feeling is reflected in the following responses:

> I was really disappointed. I was mad because it wasn't happening the way I would like. I just expected more. I expected him to be different—not to be that way. (28-year-old female, married 4 years)

> He was so different than when we first got married. And then I got pregnant so quickly—it was unplanned. We had been so close—emotionally and physically—and then he changed totally. (32-year-old female, married 7 years)

> I was definitely disappointed in being married to her. I had made a mistake the first time. I don't know how I got into it the second time, but it happened. (31-year-old male, married 3 years)

In general, these disaffected spouses were not individuals who hastily got married at a young age or after a brief courtship. The average age at marriage was approximately 24 years, and the average length of time they had known their spouse before marriage was a little more than 2 years. Sixteen percent of the respondents had been previously married. But the disappointment expressed by these spouses sounded as though they were caught by surprise, tricked or cheated by love. What were these people expecting from their partners? Were their expectations too high, unrealistic, or unachievable?

When describing feelings of disillusionment, spouses often made a comparison of the partner before and after the marriage. They emphasized radical and inexplicable changes in the partner's behavior after the wedding. What had changed, for the most part, was not the partner but the respondent's perception of their partner. Beck (1988) describes the change in perception as switching lenses through which one sees the partner. Negative labels are now attached to the same characteristics that had been previously described in glowing terms. The partner's easygoing manner and free spirit is now described as "flakiness," and what was viewed as playfulness is now considered childishness (Beck, 1988). The following respondent's description of his wife illustrates this changing perception of her behavior after marriage:

> I realized her exaggerations before we were married, but they were never destructive. I accepted it and thought it was part of her bubbling, enthusiastic personality. (39-year-old male, married 17 years)

Once perceived as a woman with a "bubbling, enthusiastic personality," this respondent relabled the same behavior as overemotional and destructive. This change in perspective is critical in relationships because it results in a change in feelings. As Beck (1988) further explains, "When they perceived each other in positive terms, they felt love; when they devalued each other, they felt resentment" (pp. 28–29).

The concept of *illusionary intimacy* provides one explanation for this change in perception of the partner (Kersten & Kersten, 1988). During courtship feelings of closeness are experienced, but they are perpetuated by romanticism and idealistic perceptions of the partner and the relationship. The individual is viewing the partner as he or she would like him or her to be, and the feelings of closeness are enhanced by this idealized perception of what the partner is like. Illusionary intimacy is also supported by the fact that many individuals are on their best behavior throughout the dating period. Once they are married and living together, it becomes more difficult to hide negative attributes. "Not only does the situation of living together make it more difficult to gloss over such negative characteristics, but also the persons themselves may feel that they have the 'right' to relax their self-presentations and let some of the more negative characteristics manifest themselves" (Berger & Roloff, 1982, p. 181). Thus, spouses feel disappointed and deceived as they contrast the dating behavior with the married behavior.

This distorted view of the partner during the couple's courtship may also be "need-related" (Graziano & Musser, 1982). Because the person has particular needs for the relationship to continue, there is a "narrowing of attention and an increase in need-related cognitions" (p. 90). According to Graziano and Musser, "since needs may induce both need-related thoughts and the selection of a particular schema, we would anticipate that needs would lead to 'distortions' (i.e., polarized attitudes and affects)" (p. 90). These authors suggest further that the distortions are more likely to occur during the initiation period than during the maintenance period of a relationship because the primary purpose of distortion is to *begin* a sequence of behaviors. Once marital vows are exchanged and commitment to the institution of marriage is made, spouses are no longer in the initiation phase but move into the maintenance phase. They no longer have to work to attain their partner's love—they have already achieved this goal. When the relationship is established, the distortion is no longer necessary because the initial desire or need to have a relationship has been met.

Distortions may also be more common in the beginning of a relationship because they have not been subjected to the reality constraints of an ongoing relationship (Graziano & Musser, 1982). But as reality sets in, disillusionment with the partner occurs. Thus, the disappointment that is experienced after marriage stems from a combination of the partner's behavior actually changing (he or she no longer needs to be on best behavior) and the disappearance of a need-related distortion of the partner that had been functional for the initiation of the relationship.

During this initial phase of disaffection, disillusionment and disappointment were often juxtaposed with optimism about the future of their relationship. Note the sense of hope in the following responses:

> I've committed myself for life with this person. And that somewhere deep down I felt that everything will eventually be okay. We could always see a marriage counselor if it got to that point. He was going to change. He was going to see that I loved him so much. . . . I knew in my mind that if I worked hard enough, everything would be okay; this was going to be a good fruitful loving marriage. (30-year-old female, married 4 years)

> I tried to approach it with an open mind. The problems in the marriage itself do not seem to be insurmountable. If she and I could approach it from a reasonable basis, the problem can be solved. (39-year-old male, married 17 years)

In general, respondents were not contemplating leaving the marriage during this first phase of disaffection. Problems and negative feelings had not escalated to the point of wanting to escape the marriage. Spouses were hopeful about the future. This hope and future orientation kept them involved in and committed to the marital relationship.

However, it is noteworthy that a little more than one third of the respondents (35%) were at least thinking about the consequences of staying versus leaving the marriage. A typical comment was, "I thought of leaving but you just don't get divorced after one year of marriage." Thus, the option of leaving, at least for some respondents, appeared to be a fleeting thought, but not an idea that was seriously entertained at this point in the process of disaffection.

Attempts to Change the Marriage

I asked the disaffected spouses what they had done in response to the problems described during this early phase of their disaffection. Had they taken actions to resolve some of their marital problems?

Or had they passively awaited the disillusionment to grow and their love to deteriorate further? According to most respondents, actions had been taken regarding the marital problems experienced during the first phase of disaffection. While the respondents reported problem-solving actions throughout all of the phases of disaffection, during this initial phase, more so than during other phases of disaffection, respondents focused much of their effort on attempts to please their partners.

> I tried to be more the perfect wife. To go home from work and bake a pie so that I could put a piece in his lunch. Basically providing him with the same home he had when he lived with his parents. (42-year-old female, married 24 years)

> I tried to get him as involved as I could. We went to Lamaze and I tried to get him to do the exercises. I tried to keep in shape for him and please him by staying the same. (28-year-old female, married 4 years)

> I would always agree with his suggestions—whether I thought they were wrong or not, I would always agree. (26-year-old female, married 6 years)

> I changed my interests so that they were more acceptable to my husband. For example, he practiced a strict religion which prohibited dancing and rock music, so I gave up these things. I just let that stuff out of our lives for a really long time. I just kinda accepted those things being gone. I used to dance with a dance partner, and I accepted that that part of my life was gone. After awhile I just accepted all those changes. (28-year-old female, married 4 years)

A sense of burden, responsibility, and self-blame were reflected in the voices of these women as they described the lengths to which they attempted to take care of the partner and relationship. When asked about sources of the problem, 59% of the respondents blamed themselves for the problems. The woman quoted above who tried pleasing her husband by baking him a pie stated, "I never blamed him. I felt the only problem was that I couldn't adjust. I was creating the problem." Another woman explained:

> I thought I wasn't a good wife. I thought I was doing something wrong. I couldn't figure out what it was. But he had blamed me. He'd get mad, and he'd say "Oh, you've made me mad, it's your fault." And I just believed that it was my fault. (26-year-old female, married 8 years)

Assuming responsibility for the problems meant they could also assume the responsibility for their solutions. The attempt to solve the marital problems was a more likely response for the women in my sample than for the men. Other research has found that women are more likely than men to take an active role in responding to marital problems (Rusbult, 1987). The strong cultural prescriptions for women to be caretakers of their relationships encourage these attempts to please the spouse and make the relationship better. There is a growing body of literature (Chodorow, 1978; Gilligan, 1982; Jack, 1991; Jordan, Kaplan, Miller, Stiver, & Surrey, 1991) that emphasizes the primacy of connection or relatedness to a woman's sense of self and well-being. This need for connection along with cultural prescriptions to be caretakers of relationships can result in desperate attempts to fix the relationship when it goes awry.

The danger of these "pleasing behaviors" is that they set up a pattern in the marriage that communicates to the partner of the pleaser that if there are problems in the marriage the pleaser will take responsibility for them. During later phases of disaffection, after repeated unsuccessful attempts at solving the problems on their own, many of the disaffected spouses concluded that the non-disaffected partner also needed to change in order to improve the marital relationship. At this later point in the process, the pleasers began to feel that the fate of the relationship was beyond their own control. However, the nondisaffected partner was often still expecting their pleasing spouse to take care of the relationship.

Some disaffected spouses (20%) chose not to express complaints to their partners but instead withdrew from them. Again, consistent with the earlier observation that women were more likely to respond actively to relationship problems, I found that many of the male respondents chose a passive response, as illustrated by the following:

> I never discussed it or brought it up to her. Well, maybe in the heat of an argument there may be something that was said. One of the problems was that my wife and I could not sit and discuss anything—really totally talk about it. (47-year-old male, married 25 years)

> I might have said something in general to my drinking buddies. But as far as sitting down and being open to someone, I don't think I did that too often. (43-year-old male, married 21 years)

> I spent nights out to avoid her. I tried to stretch the work as long as possible before coming home. (38-year-old male, married 2 years)

Unlike the previous female responses, these responses do not convey a sense of responsibility for the relationship problems or of self-blame. On the contrary, they communicate an avoidance of problems and neglect of the relationship.

Reactions of the Nondisaffected Partner

Did the nondisaffected partners recognize the marital dissatisfactions? Were *they* making attempts to change? Although the partners were not interviewed, I did ask the disaffected spouses for their perceptions of their husband's or wife's behavior. The question about the partner's behavior followed the question about the respondent's actions during the particular phase of disaffection. While these responses were based on one spouse's perception and may be somewhat biased, they shed some light on what appeared to be the couple's interaction during times of stress and conflict in their marriage.

During the first phase of disaffection, a majority of the respondents (69%) reported that their partner was making no changes and even that he or she denied that there were any problems in the marriage. Two other common responses "disagreed/argued" and "withdrawal" also gave the impression that the partners were refusing to acknowledge or face the problems in the marriage. There were a variety of ways that the partners demonstrated their reluctance to deal with marital dissatisfaction, as illustrated by the following responses:

> She was defensive and made excuses. I think that's one of the main things that bothers me about this relationship that she accepts responsibility for nothing. It's always "somebody else's fault" or "I didn't have any control in the situation." (38-year-old male, married 2 years)

> He would not listen. He said I was nagging him and that I was making mountains out of molehills, overreacting, I was an overprotective mother. I had Protective Services calling me to ask about the children's bruises. I wasn't overreacting. (31-year-old female, married 3 years)

> Her [the partner's] attitude was "I just have to be strong and he'll get over this." I called it the ostrich complex—she would put her head in the sand and wait for the storm to blow over.... She would wait for it to blow over. (47-year-old male, married 20 years)

> He started to call me "woman libber." He just attributed it to the fact that I was easily influenced. That's not true. And he always minimized it. To him it was just a phase, like a child going through a phase. (42-year-old female, married 24 years)

It is apparent that these respondents perceived that their feelings and concerns were not heard or taken seriously by the nondisaffected partner. The disaffected spouse lacked a real voice in the marriage. Moreover, the partner's invalidating the spouse's feelings and denying problems in the marriage seemed to lead to the disaffected spouse questioning the legitimacy of his or her own complaints with the marriage. Having a third party to confirm one's reality (as illustrated by the response of the second respondent above) assisted the spouses in deciding that their complaints were valid. But without the third party, the disaffected spouse may continue to question his or her own feelings and perception of the marriage. Convinced by the nondisaffected partner that "everything is okay," the disaffected spouses could begin to ignore or suppress any feelings of dissatisfaction.

The nondisaffected partner's denial of marital problems can also contribute to the unilateral nature of disaffection. As long as dissatisfaction or conflict in the marriage is not affecting the partner in any negative way, the partner does not recognize any need to change. The partner continues to be content and committed to the relationship, while the disaffected individual quietly contemplates his or her unhappiness and disappointment in the relationship.

Some of the respondents (39%) reported that their nondisaffected partners made attempts to please them. But because these pleasing behaviors frequently occurred after a blowup or some other type of serious incident provoked by the partner, these actions were often interpreted by the disaffected spouse as appeasing and placating. These actions by the partner appeared similar to the extremely kind and contrite loving behavior of a batterer after an acute battering incident as described in a cycle of violence (Walker, 1979). This behavior usually lures the spouse back into the relationship and into a sense of hope that the partner is truly sorry and will not do it again.

> The next day he bought me flowers. He never talked about the physical stuff, but he said something about the fight we had and that he was sorry. (35-year-old female, married 5 years)

I was a patient in the Center, and it was like he was taking care of me. And he got real nice, and he was going out of his way to please me, except in that one area. He would get mad if you said he was an alcoholic or try to blame him for any of the problems. But otherwise he seemed to go out of his way. (48-year-old female, married 25 years)

He did some physical things to help [baby care and house-cleaning]. But as far as talking to me, he really didn't help in that way. (53-year-old female, married 21 years)

Again, what was missing from these "pleasing" attempts by the partner was the sense of real listening to the spouse. This is especially apparent in this last account. While the respondent's husband was eager to "do" something to mend the problem, for over 20 years what this woman really wanted was for her husband to talk with her.

The predominant perception of the disaffected spouses was that their partners were not making the desired changes. Even when changes were made, they were often short-lived. A typical example of a short-lived change was a substance abusing partner who would stop taking drugs, only to start up after a few weeks. After a pattern of short-lived changes, respondents voiced that they often were suspicious of any lasting changes.

Coping Strategies

Marital stress can take its toll on a spouse's well-being, as well as the well-being of the relationship. During our discussion of each phase of the disaffection process, I asked respondents how they were coping with their marital distress. Respondents reported that a wide range of coping strategies were being used to deal with marital doubts and growing disillusionment. During the initial phase of disaffection, avoidant and passive types of coping strategies were most frequently used. More than half of the respondents (53%)

reported that they kept silent; about one third (35%) stated that they employed denial as a means of coping.

> I denied a lot of what he was doing, a lot of things I was feeling. I kept trying to tell myself it was my imagination—a pregnant woman's anxiety. . . . I also kept busy. I worked full time during my pregnancy to try to keep my mind off it. And when I wasn't working, I had my aerobics class. I kept busy so that I didn't have to think about it. (23-year-old female, married 3 years)

> I just kept telling myself it would get better. Basically denial, I guess. (30-year-old male, married 7 years)

> I was pretty passive. I cried. But I didn't do anything active to cope with it. . . . I kept things inside. (35-year-old female, married 5 years)

> I would take long walks and spend a lot of time with my mother but didn't talk to her about my marriage. (46-year-old female, married 30 years)

> I always kept all my emotions inside. I just went about my daily business—I worked and came home and took care of the house. . . . I held a lot in. (26-year-old female, married 7 years)

> I would try to keep peace. I would just bury it. I ignored it. (42-year-old female, married 24 years)

> I kept it inside. I didn't have anyone to talk to. (36-year-old female, married 15 years)

This last woman reported keeping things inside until her eleventh year of disaffection when she finally talked with a counselor.

It is apparent that many of these disaffected spouses suffered in silence. Were they without any social support? Probably not. It is more likely that they were reluctant to admit marital problems to friends and family. Because the majority of respondents had experienced marital doubts during the first year of the marriage, it may have been too embarrassing to these spouses to admit dissatisfaction so early in the marriage. In addition, there is a taboo in our culture that discourages spouses from talking about their marriages. This "intermarital taboo" states that married couples cannot talk openly to each other about their marriages (Mace & Mace, 1986). Unfortunately, because of this taboo, couples do not have the chance to share with one another the stresses of married life and the possible ways to cope effectively with them (Mace & Mace, 1986).

When the respondents did risk revealing their marital discontent to someone, they usually chose a family member or close friend as a confidant—rarely were professionals used at this stage. This tendency to avoid involvement of professional people outside of the dyadic unit is consistent with other studies on relationship breakdown that have shown that people are reluctant to involve support from others until the later stages of the breakdown (Duck, 1982; Vaughan, 1986).

Some respondents resorted to more self-punitive types of coping such as overeating, excessive sleeping, working, or shopping, substance abuse, or suicide attempts.

A lot of times I was hiding my problems in the bottle. I was quite a heavy drinker for 20 years. . . . When I was drinking I really didn't care what happened around the house, and if I wasn't drinking then perhaps if she was picky, I would say something. But if I was drinking, I'd just ignore it. . . . I was definitely drinking to escape from the problems. (43-year-old male, married 21 years)

I ate and I gained weight. There was an inverse correlation between my weight and my love for my wife. (48-year-old male, married 13 years)

At that time I was planning suicide too. I was having suicidal thoughts—I had had suicidal thoughts before but these suicidal thoughts were directly connected with getting away from this problem—solving this problem by committing suicide, getting out of the marriage. (53-year-old female, married 21 years)

I started to shop. . . . It would take my mind off it. It would give me something to do. It would keep me from getting depressed. It made me feel that at least someone was doing something nice for me—even if it was just myself. And in the meantime I just totally screwed up the financial picture. (32-year-old female, married 4 years)

This last response illustrates how these ineffective types of coping behaviors were not only destructive to the self but could harm the relationship as well. As ineffective coping strategies, such as excessive drinking, eating, shopping, are employed by the dis-affected spouse, more distress in the marital relationship and more marital dissatisfaction are likely to occur. A downward spiral of the relationship follows.

Summary

Table 2.2 summarizes the feelings, thoughts, and behaviors of the beginning phase of marital disaffection as distilled from the data from my study. This beginning phase was characterized by feelings of anger, hurt, and disillusionment by the respondents. Disillusionment involved the reduction of both idealism and high expectations for the marriage. It did not necessarily mean that the spouses were

TABLE 2.2 Characteristics of Phase I: Disappointment

Feelings:	Anger, hurt, disillusionment
Thoughts:	Awareness of partner's flaws; thinking that marriage is not turning out as expected; assuming responsibility for relationship
Behaviors:	Attempts are made to solve marital problems unilaterally; person tries to please partner; avoidant and passive coping strategies (silence, denial) are used

disaffected and that love and affection had significantly diminished. However, the perception of the partner was changing. Spouses were using different lenses in viewing their partner. Flaws that had been previously glossed over were now quite apparent. What were previously defined as positive traits were now relabeled as negative.

While disappointed in the marriage, the disaffecting spouses were not contemplating leaving the marriage at this time but were holding on to the hope that the marital relationship would improve. In general, the disaffecting spouses assumed responsibility for marital problems during this phase. They tried to change the marriage by pleasing and accommodating the nondisaffected partner—trying to be a "perfect" spouse, in the words of one respondent. Assuming the responsibility for the marital problems was also reinforced by the seeming denial and indifference to any marital concerns by the nondisaffected partner.

In coping with their marital dissatisfactions during this early phase, respondents were primarily keeping silent and denying the gravity of the marital situation. Seeking support and help from their friends, family, or a helping professional rarely occurred.

While most spouses experience some disappointment or disillusionment with their marital partners, for many it does not lead to the experience of marital disaffection. However, some spouses, like the respondents in this study, continue down the path of disaffection. In the next chapter, we examine what happens to move spouses along this road.

Note

1. For the sake of clarity in distinguishing between the disaffected respondents and their partners (who were not interviewed), I will refer to the respondents as "spouse" or "spouses" and to the partners of the respondents "partner" or "partners."

T·H·R·E·E

Between Disappointment and Disaffection

I was desperately hoping that somebody would run him over. I was fantasizing that he would get hit by a truck somewhere, someday soon.

(30-year-old female, married 4 years)

Feelings of Anger

As the spouses continued down the path of marital disaffection, the feeling of disillusionment dissipated and anger increased. The disaffected spouse was no longer shocked or surprised by the partner's behavior. Whereas about one half of the respondents reported feeling disappointed in their partner during the beginning phase, only 22% were reporting this feeling during the middle phase. They stated that by this time they were even expecting their partner to behave in certain negative ways. But expecting this behavior did not mean the respondents were less upset or angry with their partner. Reports of anger not only increased in frequency but also in intensity, as exemplified by the following poignant statements:

> I had fantasies of killing him.... After I heard about the woman in Michigan putting her husband's bed on fire, I fantasized setting our bed on fire and burning my husband up.... I didn't have any thoughts of getting out of the marriage in any other way, but I had thoughts of hating him, killing him, and burning him up. (53-year-old female, married 4 years)

I never had thoughts of leaving the marriage. I never knew I had a choice. . . . All of a sudden I realized, what am I doing here? . . . I wished he would die. (54-year-old female, married 36 years)

I could have killed him if I had the right vehicle. I didn't want to be around him—I wanted to just get out of his life. (27-year-old female, married 4 years)

Upon hearing about her husband's extramarital affair, one woman described her feelings of shock and anger:

It was a friend of my husband who came to me and told me. As soon as the words came out of his mouth, as soon as I realized and heard with my own ears that my husband was living with someone and had already had this girlfriend for months, I really want to say for the record I know what it means to have your blood turn cold. I know that feeling. I felt like I fell out of love. . . . I have told people that for the past year. I fell out of love immediately. It was gone. He was a stranger to me—gut hate. . . . Then I immediately went to an attorney and filed for divorce without even discussing it with him. . . . I wanted to kill him. No, I wanted to hurt him. . . . Boy was I a fool. . . . I let myself be duped. Wasted time. I wasted 3 years of my life. And it's all his fault. (30-year-old female, married 4 years)

These actions and feelings may appear quite extreme, but this was not the first time respondents had had to deal with some break of trust or some kind of a crisis. The process of disaffection may have been progressing for years, and this was just one more crisis that added to their accumulating anger.

How the disaffected spouses expressed their anger ranged from very subtle actions to quite obvious acts of hostility. The following is an example of the former:

> If my wife said something or did something that upset me . . . I would not let her know about it. . . . I would not say anything to acknowledge it. . . . Quite often there have been things done or said that I thought should not be done or said, but due to my not wanting to hurt other people's feelings, I'm not assertive. . . . My wife tells me I'm sarcastic a lot. . . . I give in to try to avoid an argument—that's happened throughout most of the marriage. (43-year-old male, married 21 years)

In contrast, another woman expressed her anger in a more overt way when her husband chose a military career against her wishes.

> I got mad at him, and I bleached all his uniforms. I was just going to give him no support. I was going to try to make him the worst military man they had in the whole world. If he wasn't going to get out, I was going to try to have him kicked out. . . . I was going to do whatever I had to do. I wasn't going to be dumped for the military. (28-year-old female, married 4 years)

What the last two respondents had in common was the inability to confront their partner directly with their dissatisfactions; instead they used passive–aggressive behaviors to express it. Unless the partner could decipher clues about his or her spouse's anger and directly discuss the anger with the spouse, the partner was likely to participate in this collusion to avoid conflict. Many of the disaffected spouses were committed to "keep peace" at all costs in order to maintain the relationship—even if it meant not dealing with their marital dissatisfactions.

Feelings of Hurt

Closely related to anger, hurt was another predominant feeling experienced during this phase. The hurt appeared to stem from recurrences of the partner's negative and injurious behaviors. Often disaffected spouses interpreted these negative behaviors in a personal and intentional way, as if the partner was behaving in a way to purposefully hurt the spouse. Some respondents expressed hurt regarding feeling second to work or children in their partner's life. In general, there was a feeling of being unloved and uncared for.

> This man really doesn't love me at all. He loves himself and that is it—he was looking for someone to love him. I don't think he loves me. He was looking for someone to take care of him. . . . You keep hoping, but eventually you see it and say this is over. I went through a lot of grieving. Something had died. It was real sad. (31-year-old female, married 2 years)

> Maybe what I have to say isn't important. Maybe what I have to say is frivolous and emotional, and I'm not being rational. Maybe that is wrong. . . . Then I'd think, "Wait a minute, I am important. Just because I don't handle situations the same as you doesn't make me any less. You're treating me less because I'm more emotional. No, I'm not less than you are. I'm different than you are. I handle my life different. I think differently; I think with my heart rather than my head. That doesn't make me less of a person." (36-year-old female, married 15 years)

Upon hearing about his wife's unfaithfulness during his military duty, one respondent expressed his hurt with the following:

> At first I thought, "I'm a fool to put that much trust in somebody. . . . I was let down." It wasn't *what* she had done that really got to me. What got to me was the fact that she lied to me for the whole time. That was what I was angry and hurt about. (30-year-old male, married 10 years)

While in the first phase of disaffection there had been some doubts about their marriage, the respondents overall were quite hopeful and still cared about their partner. However, during the middle phase they started to question whether they still loved their partner, and the notion of "falling out of love" was entering their awareness. Until this time the respondents may not have used the phrase "falling out of love" or even recognized it as such. Interestingly, they were now viewing their relationship and feelings about it as a process—not as a static, isolated event but a sequence of events producing their current feelings about the marriage.

> It's such a gradual thing, I don't think I ever wanted to admit that I wasn't in love with him. . . . But romantically I didn't want him to touch me, and we fought continuously. And I preferred not to be around him unless we were with a group of people, and then we couldn't fight. I think all of a sudden one day I realized, "I'm just not in love with this man." (34-year-old female, married 12 years)

> What is going on is very unfair. I had put up with so much from him and was trying to keep things going. This is getting to be the ultimate thing—I'm not going to choose between him and the children. He felt that if I loved him, there's no question that I would agree with everything he said. . . . His actions had already pushed away my feelings for him. And I was struggling to stay in love with him. (43-year-old female, married 9 years)

> At that time I was thinking that I didn't know if I loved him. I had lived with this so long. I didn't know what real love was. . . . If he left me, I wouldn't die. (46-year-old female, married 30 years)

Whereas in the previous phase it was easy to dismiss the problems and hurts as aberrations, now they were recurring, not easily forgiven or forgotten, and chipping away at the respondents' love. Accordingly, apathy also became increasingly evident during this phase. None of the respondents reported feelings of apathy during the beginning phase, but during the middle phase 16% of the respondents reported it—a small number, but an indication that love was beginning to die. The last quote, in particular, gives a sense of a heart already turned cold.

Negative Evaluation of Partner

The thoughts accompanying these feelings of anger and hurt focused on the negative traits of the partners—their controlling behavior, drinking, lying, irresponsibility, and so on. About 70% of the respondents reported that they were focusing on the negative traits of their partner during this phase. This concentration on negative traits contrasts starkly with an earlier time when the spouses were falling in love and *rarely* saw anything wrong with their partner. As relationships become troubled, views of the partners change and spouses relate to their partner in terms of their negative traits. As spouses become increasingly unhappy, they start to dwell on and even exaggerate their partner's flaws (Vaughan, 1986).

Why do spouses shift their cognitive focus from positive traits of the partner to negative traits? Two explanations may account for this tendency. First, the *figure–ground* explanation states that "since persons expect to experience good things in their everyday lives, including the actions of others, when a person displays negative attributes, these characteristics stand out and assume an inordinate weight in the overall impression formed" (Berger & Roloff, 1982, p. 180). Remember that many spouses had a distorted positive perspective of their partner in the beginning of the relationship—especially during courtship. However, with time the spouses began to recognize their partner's flaws, and these contrasted sharply with the previous idealization of the partner and became more salient to the disaffecting spouses.

A second explanation, based on the concept of *vigilance,* suggests that in order to avoid further hurt, persons may become more sensitive to the potential hurtful actions of others and be less sensitive to the positive actions of others (Berger & Roloff, 1982). This cognitive process appears to be a survival mechanism in dealing with potential dangers posed by other people. In an attempt to protect oneself from further hurt by a partner's actions, one becomes more sensitive to and cognizant of the partner's negative behaviors. Of course, in reality, this vigilance may not protect the person from further hurt. For example, constantly thinking about a partner's untrustworthy behaviors may not prevent them from occurring again. But to dismiss and ignore these behaviors may result in a greater disappointment if they do happen again. More important to the process of disaffection, though, this vigilance results in the accentuation of negative behaviors in the mind of the spouse, and eventually the negative behaviors overshadow any positive actions of the partner.

This focus on negative behaviors of the partner has serious implications for any attempts at stopping the progression of the process of disaffection. When the partner's negative behaviors predominate, it may be even more difficult to change the person's feelings toward the partner. Although the partner may promise to change and, in fact, does change, these changes may not be enough to overcome the deleterious effects of the partner's remaining negative behaviors (Berger & Roloff, 1982). The negative behaviors are not only more salient than the positive behaviors but another process is also occurring: The spouse may see a consistency of the behaviors over time that leads the spouse to conclude that these negative behaviors are part of the partner's personality and are likely to be immutable. Whereas earlier in the process a negative behavior may have been attributed to a factor outside the couple or be seen as a situational factor, now it is viewed as part of the partner's disposition. Regardless of the explanation for it, focus on the negative behaviors of a partner has a deteriorating effect on a close relationship. It creates a type of tunnel vision through which the spouse looks only at the flaws of the partner and begins to doubt whether the partner can change.

At the end of the process, these same negative thoughts may serve a different purpose for those disaffected spouses who decide to leave the marriage. By focusing on the negative behaviors, the disaffected spouse can be developing his or her story for leaving the person and thus "begin to create something to leave behind"

(Vaughan, 1986, p. 44). The disaffected spouse convinces himself or herself that dissolution is warranted and indeed justifiable. Because the respondents had not reached a decision to leave during this phase of disaffection, it appeared that they were not yet focusing on the negative behaviors to justify leaving.

Assessing Rewards and Costs of the Marriage

Evaluating rewards and costs of the marriage was a common cognitive activity throughout the disaffection process. However, there was an increase in these thoughts during the middle phase, when 60% of the respondents reported its occurrence. Basic to the development of an intimate relationship is the idea that its perceived rewards outweigh its perceived costs (Thibaut & Kelley, 1959). People are particularly mindful of the rewards and costs of a relationship during the courtship period because they are making decisions about the continuation of the relationship. Similarly, during the breakdown of a relationship, individuals are carefully examining the reward–cost ratio as they are making decisions regarding the relationship's potential for change or the possibility of its dissolution. The following response exemplifies this assessment of rewards and costs during the middle phase:

> Do I really love her? I know I care about her; she was a very good friend of mine. I considered her on that basis, but I really questioned in my mind if I really loved her. She wasn't what I wanted, but does everybody get exactly what they want in a relationship? I've got a lot of good things here. Basically just trying to weigh things out. (30-year-old male, married 7 years)

Love, status, money, support, security, and validation are the types of rewards desired in a close relationship (Levinger, 1979). Costs of staying in a relationship may involve one's time, energy, and various other expenditures (Levinger, 1979). During the breakdown of a relationship there is a drastic shift in perceived rewards or costs.

When relationships are on the up-swing, mutual rewards are believed to be highly probable and thoughts of costs are suppressed; later, during disenchantment one or both partners find the old rewards less probable, and unanticipated costs are now discovered. In some cases, the eventual costs existed from the beginning but neither partner had wanted to see them; in other instances, the components of attraction change markedly over the course of time. (Levinger, 1979, p. 41)

The spouse's view of rewards and costs—even regarding the same behavior—may change during the course of the marriage. For example, the continual care and attention given by a partner may have been perceived as rewarding in the beginning of the relationship but later is viewed as smothering or manipulative.

Did the respondents evaluate the reward–cost ratio of their marriages even before the disaffection process began? In other words, when a spouse is satisfied with the marriage, will he or she still be monitoring the reward–cost ratio of the marriage? Studies of exchange theory and intimate relationships suggest that couples do have a sense of equitable exchange of rewards and that happy couples perceive the rewards to be greater than the costs (Scanzoni & Scanzoni, 1988; Walster, Walster, & Berscheid, 1978). However, marital exchange is not as carefully monitored among the happy spouses (Levinger, 1979). One potential signal of a relationship's downturn is when either partner worries about mutual equity or the fairness of the marital exchange (Levinger, 1979, 1983).

Certain personality variables, situations, and types of relationships may result in an individual being especially concerned with equity or inequity in a relationship (Hatfield, Traupmann, Sprecher, Utne, & Hay, 1985). As yet there has been little research on how personality and relationship variables impact a person's monitoring of the reward–cost ratio. When there are abrupt and obvious changes in what is being exchanged, inequity and injustice may be especially salient (Leventhal, 1980). For example, take a case where both spouses are working and one loses his or her job. The spouse who is totally supporting the family may begin to pay attention to rewards and costs in the relationship more than before. Any significant shift of the reward–cost ratio—whether it be in money, status, physical attractiveness, support, and so on—may lead spouses to question the balance of rewards and costs in their relationship (Hatfield et al., 1985) and perhaps wonder if they deserve better.

Another reason for the cognitive focus on rewards and costs in the marriage is their potency in a close relationship. The costs or punishments imposed by an intimate can be more powerful than punishments imposed by other people.

> For example, if a stranger at a party loudly announces that I am a selfish bore, I lose little; I can dismiss his words as those of a creep who doesn't really know what kind of person I am. But if my best friend were to tell me the same thing, I would be crushed—she knows me, and still thinks that! As Aronson (1970) succinctly put it: "Familiarity may breed reward, but it also breeds the capacity to hurt." (Walster et al., 1978, p. 149)

Thus, it is difficult for spouses to gloss over hurts and costs incurred by the partner. Rather, these hurts can become the focus of attention, and they fester if not forgiven and forgotten.

Finally, the concern with equity may depend on the spouse's view of his or her alternatives. The person who sees no alternatives to the relationship may not be very concerned with the equity or inequity of the relationship, whereas the individual who perceives attractive alternatives to the current relationship can better afford to attend to the inequity in it (Hatfield et al., 1985). However, I found in my interviews that spouses without perceived alternatives attended to the inequity in their marriages, thus making them feel even more trapped in the relationship. Not only were they in an unfair relationship but they could not perceive any alternatives that were better than staying in their marriage. Often they would rationalize their staying in the inequitable relationship by focusing on barriers to leaving it, such as the consequences of divorce on children, the lack of financial security, and religious/moral obligations.

Thoughts about Leaving the Partner

What had previously been a fleeting thought—leaving—was now being considered more seriously. Some respondents spent an inordinate amount of time contemplating the option of leaving the marriage. Approximately 40% reported during the middle phase that they were trying to decide whether to stay in or to leave the marriage. Often specific barriers to leaving, such as children, finances, or religion, were mentioned. The following response is an example of what a respondent was saying to herself as she contemplated this dilemma of staying versus leaving:

> Now I'm going to be done with this. What's going to go on in my life? It's time to make a decision. I'm going to be 30 years old when I'm done with this. I've got to either pull this marriage together to make it what I believe it could be or it's gotta stop. If it's never going to be what I want, it's time for me to leave this relationship. I've given 10 years of my life to it. I'm 30 years old. I didn't have a family, I didn't have a home, I didn't have a lot of the things I wanted and now was the time to make it what it should be or end it. But I hadn't realized how sucked into alcohol he had become—how his addiction had grown. Because he was able to hide it from me very effectively.
>
> I really spent all those hours alone thinking about what I wanted to do. Did I want to leave him? Did I want to have a relationship with my brother-in-law, who I had always been really close to? Did I want to meet someone totally different? What did I want to do with my life? And I really came to think that I wanted to put closeness back in my marriage. . . . I knew that he had to do something about the drinking. (31-year-old female, married 11 years)

Although she was spending much time thinking about leaving, this woman was not ready to give up on her husband or marriage yet. Despite the mounting doubts, she was still hopeful that he would change and that closeness would return to the marriage. Unlike this respondent, the next woman focused more on the barriers to leaving rather than actually improving the marriage. Although married for only a few years, barriers to leaving had already been built. Hers is a voice of resignation:

> I couldn't get divorced. I had been married before when very young, when I was 18. . . . That's why I was so damned adamant that this marriage was going to work. I'm not going to be a twice statistic. Also I had the pride from the family to deal with on my own. Also his children had just gone through a divorce with him and his ex-wife, and I kept telling them, "Your daddy and I are not going to be apart." . . . That is probably the biggest thing that kept me from seriously considering getting a divorce. (30-year-old female, married 4 years)

Another respondent resigned to the marriage cited similar barriers to leaving:

> I had made my mind up that I couldn't go anyplace. That I would just have to live with it until the kids were out of school or of an age where they could accept things. I was very close to the boys. We did a great many things with them. I just felt it would be devastating for them. And financially it would have put a bind on us. I was stuck. (47-year-old male, married 25 years)

From the beginning of their disaffection, the respondents were thinking about the barriers to ending the relationship. Barriers such as social network pressure, religious norms, and the consequences of divorce on children served to keep the person in the marriage. However, in the beginning of the disaffection process there were still attractions or rewards within the marriage that produced positive emotions and kept the couple together. As love and any positive feelings began to die, barriers may have been the only factors keeping the marriage together. Coined an "empty shell" marriage, Goode (1961) describes this kind of union as lacking emotional substance and joy:

> The atmosphere is without laughter or fun, and a sullen gloom pervades the household. Members do not discuss their problems or experiences with each other, and communication is kept to a minimum. . . . Their rationalization for avoiding a divorce is, on the part of one or both, sacrifice for the children, neighborhood respectability, and a religious conviction that divorce is morally wrong . . . . The hostility in such a home is great, but arguments focus on the small issues, not the large ones. Facing the latter would, of course, lead directly to separation or divorce, but the couple has decided that staying together overrides other values, including each other's happiness and the psychological health of their children. (pp. 441–442)

A male respondent described his empty shell marriage with the following:

> I think the situation has gotten into the business of the kids and getting them through college. Work started taking up more time. So it continued as a partnership type of arrangement without any real emotional kind of thing about it.
>
> If there was a way to get out of the thing, maybe I'd like to get out. On the other hand, I say, "Now at this point in time—unless I have some place to go, why bother?" I mean, we don't fight. I do what I want to do. I go where I want to go. She basically does what she wants to do, goes where she wants to go. She does a half-way decent job of taking care of the house.
>
> I guess I have to relate it to the old cliche—"jumping from the frying pan into the fire." Am I going to be better off without or with her. I don't particularly want to live by myself. The situation is not uncomfortable—in the sense I'm not restricted anymore than what's reasonable. If I want to go to

> Georgia for a week golfing, then I go. If I want to go to Arizona for a week, then I go. If I want to take off for the weekend and go fishing, then I usually go. If she wants to go to Colorado with some of her girlfriends or go skiing, she can go. . . . (62-year-old male, married 39 years)

Notice how this man (and also his wife) accommodated to the situation of an empty shell marriage. He identified some rewards—"she does a half-way decent job of taking care of the house"—and recognized the cost of loneliness if he did leave her. Also, his wife allows him to spend time with his friends while she spends time with hers. These are all explanations for staying in a devitalized marriage. There may not be many intrinsic or emotional rewards in this marriage, but the costs of staying are not too painful.

About 30% of the respondents during the middle phase were planning to end the marriage—a significant increase from only 4% in the first phase. These respondents who were planning to leave were thinking about some specific action such as looking for an apartment, applying for a job, or contacting an attorney.

Continued Efforts to Change the Marriage

About one third of the respondents reported that they hoped the marriage would work out during the middle phase. Most respondents reported similar types of efforts to make changes as they had during the beginning phase. Problem-solving attempts continued to be the most frequently cited action (63%). Just as their emotions appeared more intense during this middle phase, descriptions of the problem-solving behaviors were more direct and assertive in comparison to the previous phase.

> I told him that I was ready to leave. I wanted a divorce then. So he enrolled himself into a hospital for drug and alcohol abuse. And he got out, and he was good for 6 months. He didn't touch a drop or do any kind of drugs. And then gradually at work he started drinking a little bit. And then he started

smoking marijuana a little bit. And gradually he started going downhill again. (26-year-old female, married 7 years)

Another respondent tried desperately to get his wife into treatment for alcohol abuse.

I was trying to get her committed for alcohol inpatient treatment when she appeared before the judge on a drunk driving charge. I was communicating with physicians, counselors, and clergy to obtain enough evidence to show the judge she had a problem and needed help. (39-year-old male, married 17 years)

During this phase, respondents were no longer passively going along with what their partner wanted but were asserting their own desires and feelings. Especially for the women, a transformation from compliance and subservience to their husbands to expressing a voice of their own began during this phase. This was brought on both by an increase in the women's self-esteem and confidence and by their becoming aware of alternative ways of interacting in marriage. One woman shared the following thoughts during the middle phase of her disaffection. She had recently returned to work—an action of which her husband disapproved.

I was tired of doing always what he wanted. . . . For the first time I felt it was okay to have different ideas. I wasn't crazy. The girls I worked with were several years younger than me. . . . I could see the difference in their marriages and mine. They would do things with their husbands which to my husband would seem stupid and frivolous. (42-year-old female, married 24 years)

Another respondent found attending school to be both confidence building and liberating from her husband's domination.

When I quit that job I started to go to school. I was a sponge. I couldn't get enough. I was starved intellectually. And that bothered him [her husband] greatly. I don't know if he was insecure about getting attention from me and I couldn't give it while I was doing homework, or if it bothered him because I would be smarter than him. (30-year-old female, married 4 years)

Starting new jobs, going to school, making friends, and involvement in extracurricular activities boosted respondents' self-esteem so that they could stand up to their partner. But these activities also provided alternatives to the marriage—a means of financial, social, or emotional support if the marriage ended.

Coinciding with these more assertive behaviors was a decrease in the frequency of attempts to please the partner during the middle phase—although a fairly large number (39%) were still reporting some type of pleasing behaviors.

I continued to try to please him but probably did less of it. I was busy working and with the kids, I probably ignored him more. I was making good money. I was happy with my job. . . . By that time I had gotten used to him not being around. (26-year-old female, married 8 years)

Physical and Emotional Withdrawal

As the hurts accumulated, the disaffected spouse wanted more physical and emotional distance from the partner. Many respondents chose this alternative in order to survive in the marriage, but others used it as a strategy to change the relationship. If trying harder to please the partner was not working, why not try an opposite tactic and withdraw?

I became cold towards him—hardly talking to him and not sharing anything with him and became kinda shut up inside myself. And almost didn't even acknowledge he was even there. (53-year-old female, married 21 years)

However, when withdrawal was not producing any changes in the relationship, it was primarily a coping strategy to protect or defend oneself from further hurt—a feeling that was predominant during this phase.

> When we were together I would always find something to do—to keep myself away from him. When he wanted to sit next to me or get close to me, I would always pull away or pull back. I didn't want him to touch me. At that time I knew something was wrong. (26-year-old female, married 6 years)

> We didn't have anything to do with each other. It was the happiest time of my life. (50-year-old female, married 27 years)

The withdrawal was also on a sexual level. Understandably, it was difficult for many of the disaffecting spouses to experience much sexual interest in their partner while feeling intense anger and hurt.

> I can't make love with someone I feel frustrated with and aggravated with and tense with and would rather choke than hug. (36-year-old female, married 15 years)

Some respondents went to the extent of initiating a physical separation. Twenty percent of the respondents left for several weeks or asked their partner to leave. However, only five of the respondents reported taking some type of action to actually dissolve the marriage (consulting an attorney, looking for an apartment, saving money, filing for divorce). Although about one third of the respondents were thinking about ending their marriages during the middle phase, very few were ready to act on this thought. Again, this illustrates that much cognitive activity around an important decision such as ending a marriage can occur before the partner even has a clue that a dissolution is forthcoming.

The Partner's Reactions

Regarding the partner's behavior, respondents were reporting similar behaviors during the middle phase as they had reported in the beginning phase, namely short-lived changes and denial.

> He made changes after he went to prison. He started working, writing, calling me, he went to church—he made a complete change. I started thinking maybe things will be okay. But after prison he worked at a work center where he started smoking pot. We got in a fight, and he took off for a couple days and started drinking again. (26-year-old female, married 8 years)

Some respondents reported that in reaction to their increased assertiveness, their partner was increasing his or her control and becoming more oppositional:

> He would pull in the reins tighter . . . every time I fought back he took away one more thing. He was trying to keep me at home. (53-year-old woman, married 21 years)

> He was ranting and raving . . . venting his anger. He was being very dominating. He was very adamant in what he was going to do—no compromising. [During another later incident] [h]e was domineering—wouldn't back down on decisions he had made. He abused me emotionally. He said, "You're going to do as I say not as I do." (46-year-old female, married 30 years)

Thus, a negative reciprocity emerged as some partners reacted to the respondents' aggressive attempts at changing the marriage with more aggressive behaviors. Needless to say, these behaviors only accelerated the downward spiral of the relationship and confirmed the disaffected spouses' growing negative perceptions of their partner.

Summary

Table 3.1 summarizes the feelings, thoughts, and behaviors of the middle phase of marital disaffection as distilled from the data from my interviews. By the middle phase, disillusionment (the reduction of idealism and high expectations for marriage) had significantly dissipated, and anger intensified. The respondents were no longer shocked or surprised by their partner's behaviors, and to some extent they even expected it. Hurt also continued at the same high level as it had been experienced in the beginning phase. But in reaction to repeated hurts, the disaffected spouses responded with more assertive behaviors or withdrew to protect themselves. Spouses were no longer trying to please the partner as much as they had in the beginning phase. There was more of a sense of freedom to assert their own opinions and feelings.

The cognitive activity focused on the negative traits of the partner and the reward–cost ratio of the marriage. The oversensitivity to and vigilance of negative behaviors produced a tunnel vision effect; the respondents could no longer see their partner's positive attributes because their flaws predominated. In addition, respondents began to see these flaws as inherent to the partner's personality and likely to be permanent. While more time was spent in the calculation of the reward–cost ratio of the marital relationship to their personal happiness, most of the respondents were not ready to leave the marriage during the middle phase of marital disaffection.

TABLE 3.1 Characteristics of Phase II: Between Disappointment and Disaffection

Feelings:	Intense anger and hurt
Thoughts:	Partner's negative traits are viewed as a pattern; person evaluates the rewards and costs of marriage; person considers staying in marriage versus leaving it
Behaviors:	Person continues to attempt problem-solving but more directly confronts partner about problems; person begins physical and emotional withdrawal from the marriage

F·O·U·R

Reaching Disaffection

I don't feel any emotion. I don't like him. I dread the weekend.
I dread Friday when he's going to come home.
(54-year-old female, married 36 years)

Apathy and Indifference

Increasing distance—both physical and emotional—characterized this final phase of the process of disaffection. While the anger declined somewhat from the middle phase, apathy dramatically and significantly increased and was mentioned by approximately one-half of the respondents during the last phase. Typical expressions of the apathy experienced include the following:

> I've just put up with the same behavior so long now—I just want out because I don't see him ever changing. . . . It's too late to rekindle the feelings—I don't want to try. . . . I have no respect for him. I don't trust him. I still care what happens to him because he's in such a depressed state. But I don't believe I love him anymore because I don't miss him since I've been gone. (26-year-old female, married 7 years)

> She's worn out my feelings. I don't care what she does—just leave me alone. (30-year-old male, married 10 years)

> It's hard for me to get even a shred of affection for him. . . . I feel very angry that this has gone on so long and slowly, gradually, gradually my love for him has been worn away. And

maybe if I have a safe place to talk about how angry I've been over the years, maybe I can revive some of those good feelings for him, but I don't have many anymore. (35-year-old female, married 5 years)

I moved out for 3 days. But I can't afford to live in a hotel. . . . He threatened to commit suicide if I left. But I thought I don't give a damn, he can commit suicide, at least it would put an end to this. So in a sense there is that apathy there. I don't care what he does. (57-year-old female, married 33 years)

Really nothing. I don't care if I ever see her again. (31-year-old male, married 3 years)

I try not to talk with him. . . . I've given up on trying to make our marriage work. I know that it will never work now. So all I'm concerned about is our kids. (31-year-old female, married 5 years)

Neutral—not hatred or anger. They are not ones of revenge or hatred or anger—the way they used to be. (68-year-old male, married 36 years)

This is not worth it to me to go through this kind of aggravation and frustration. That's when I divorced him. I mean I have nothing on paper, but my feelings—the way I wanted to try to communicate with him—quit. . . . I quit talking.

Maybe married life isn't as I hoped it would be . . . maybe it isn't enjoying each other. Maybe it is just a type of live-in situation where you benefit each other financially. (36-year-old female, married 15 years)

Apathy, not hate, is the opposite of love. As Reik (1976) has stated, "The most serious enemy of love is not the hostility but the indifference that one feels toward the other" (p. 97). This experience of apathy is sometimes described as being decathected from a partner. Decathected spouses have no strong positive or negative affect regarding their partner. They describe their feelings as "those you would feel for an acquaintance" (Hagestad & Smyer,

1982, p. 174). Occasionally respondents expressed caring for their partner as a human being but not as a spouse.

> I care for him as a person. I wouldn't want nothing to happen to him. But as far as loving a person like you're suppose to love him, I just think it's just gone. . . . I want his life to be good and for him to go out and find someone who could completely satisfy him. I just want my life to be left alone. (38-year-old female, married 19 years)

Respondents stated that they experienced feelings of sorrow about the relationship and pity for their partner during this phase. A feeling of pity, which was rarely expressed by respondents during the previous phases, was now reported by a quarter of the respondents. The expression of sorrow for the partner or the relationship sounded similar to what a person might feel following a death.

> It kinda feels like she's burned her bridges. The feelings may be there, but the bridge is burned. . . . There's a certain amount of sorrow. (30-year-old male, married 10 years)

> It is very similar to the grieving process of death. I attended my first funeral during this time. . . . And all the words that were spoken by the minister I equated to my husband. . . . I let myself hurt and be sorrowful, but I think somewhere along the line I missed the anger. (30-year-old female, married 4 years)

> I feel sorry for him. I guess I got my anger out. I still believe it's his fault. (44-year-old female, married 23 years)

While respondents were feeling sorry for their partners, at this point in the disaffection process it was not producing enough guilt to keep them in the marriage. Perhaps at an earlier time they would have stayed with their partner out of a sense of guilt. But over the years, hurt and anger overshadowed the guilt.

Sometimes the sorrow revolved around the loss of a fantasy:

We won't get to be Ozzie and Harriet the way my life has turned out. (30-year-old male, married 10 years)

I don't think I really grieved over the loss of him because I think our marriage was over a long time ago and we were just living together. I grieved over the loss of all these dreams, for example, taking trips. (53-year-old female, married 21 years)

Although the disaffected spouses were describing the death of their marital relationships, very few reported being lonely. In fact, reports of loneliness decreased significantly from 33% in the middle phase to 8% in the end phase. Apparently, the disaffected spouses were now turning to others for the companionship and support that had long been lacking in their marriages. In fact, confiding in others and exposing their disaffection to others were more common activities, and they provided respondents with confirmation and validation of their feelings and perceptions about their partner.

I started to realize that other people also saw his immaturity, and others would tell me, "It's about time. We thought you could do much better than him." . . . I want to get on with my life. I felt like he was weighing me down—a cement block around my neck. I was tired of him. (32-year-old female, married 13 years)

Until disaffected spouses begin sharing their disaffection with others, they usually receive little confirmation, if any at all, of their negative perception of their partner. It is quite amazing how friends and family are eager to confirm the negative traits of the spouse when it is announced by the disaffected person that they are filing for a divorce. Earlier in the process of disaffection friends and relatives may have been encouraging the person to stay in the marriage, but by the end, they seem more supportive of the person's leave-taking. Previously feeling alone in their disaffection, the spouses now feel supported as their disaffection is validated and accepted by people around them. Duck (1988) describes a similar "social phase" in his model of relationship breakdown:

> After the partners have done some fighting—and probably even while it is still in progress—there is an important unseen element to break-up: getting the support of the surrounding network of friends, relatives, and acquaintances. It is not satisfactory merely to leave a relationship: it is important to feel justified in leaving. For this reason both partners consult friends (and relatives) for advice on the problem and for extra perspectives on the partner and their own actions (LaGaipa, 1982). The network becomes involved in relationships that are breaking up and has views about them as they spoil (McCall, 1982). It also gives support to the fighting partners, takes sides, pronounces verdicts on guilt and blame, and helps to seal the occurrence of the break-up by sanctioning the dissolution (the most obvious example being a courtroom where a divorce decree is pronounced). (p. 118)

In Duck's conceptualization of this phase, the disaffected individuals are using the social network to *justify* their decision to dissolve their marriages. Many of the respondents in my study had not yet made a definite decision to dissolve their marriage but were needing input from others in order to make the decision.

Deciding to Dissolve the Marriage

During this final phase there was a substantial increase in thoughts of ending the marriage; over twice as many respondents than in the middle phase cited this as a common thought. Many of the respondents who were thinking of ending their marriage were struggling with exactly how it could be done. Whereas some individuals were not actually taking actions to dissolve the marriage, they were at least making plans about how they might end it. For some respondents these were long-range plans:

> My youngest daughter is almost 10 years old, so I thought if I could just stick it out and make things work until she gets out

of high school. Just hang around until then. (38-year-old male, married 11 years)

I'm biding my time. I want my wife to get her master's degree. Just waiting for the opportunity and best time to leave. (47-year-old male, married 25 years)

It's all in the thinking stages right now. We're moving now and will be locked into a year's lease. So I'm thinking when the year's lease will be over is when I'll want the divorce to be final. I went and spoke to a girlfriend of mine who's a lawyer and found out some information about what you have to do. . . . I'm talking about it in more concrete terms to my girlfriends. But I don't feel I could do it now financially. Better to think about it now and act upon it later. . . . I'm not happy that I decided to stick it out for another year, but it's not practical for me to say to him, "I don't want this new apartment. I just want you to take off." There's no way I could support myself unless I had free rent somewhere. (32-year-old female, married 4 years)

Some respondents were waiting for fate to end the marriage.

A lot of times I think it would be so much simpler if she just lost control of the car, it would make it easy for me. I don't see myself staying in this, but I don't quite know how to get out at this point. (38-year-male, married 2 years)

Other respondents were for the first time thinking of ending the marriage but had no specific plans.

I didn't like my husband anymore. I couldn't think of any one thing I liked about him. I realized for the first time that maybe I have a choice—I had never considered divorce, but now I was really thinking along those lines. . . . My children have grown and what am I doing here? When I first got married, I said I would never cause my children to be unhappy through divorce. And all of a sudden I realized that they were all grown and all married but one, and they really didn't need me any longer. That there was no one I really had to answer to but myself. And one of my older sons was saying, "But what about the grandchildren, they need you—they like to come across the street to have grandma and grandpa there." And I thought why should I stay there for the few times they come across the street? . . . I just couldn't picture myself living for them. (54-year-old female, married 36 years)

For this last respondent, the barriers to divorce were getting fewer and fewer, and it was becoming more difficult for her to rationalize staying in her devitalized marriage. Some spouses, however, were resigned to staying in this type of marriage.

I'm staying in it. It's just like being in a job you don't like. You do the best you can in the situation. (62-year-old male, married 23 years)

Others were still vacillating between staying and leaving.

Sometimes I feel that I have crossed the line. I've just gotten to the point where I really don't care. I've got two choices: I can walk away from it or try to get back over to the other side of the line.

I'm not a quitter. . . I find it very difficult to be in a situation where the end of the marriage exists. Because that spells failure to me—especially with the kids.

Have you read the book *Men Who Can't Love* [Carter & Sokol, 1987]? Commitment phobic is what is discussed in this book. And the commitment phobic can't make a commitment one way or the other. And I feel like a commitment phobic at this time in the relationship. I can't make up my mind which way I want to go. It's not my style. I'm more of a decisive person. (33-year-old male, married 10 years)

Sometimes I think that as soon as the roommate leaves, I'm leaving. And then other times I think I'll wait and see if this counselor is going to help. And then I'm scared about how he will act if I leave him. Real scared. Just wondering what would happen. I think he loves me a great deal—he tries to be real affectionate. But it's like I cringe when he touches me. He tries to hold my hand when we go places, and I don't want to hold it.

I don't know what to do. I'm frightened. . . . Maybe there'll come a time when I'll leave him. I keep making excuses. First, I made the excuse that my daughter had to finish school. She finished school, and now I make the excuse about an operation. I don't have to stay for the operation, but I think that part of me wants to find some way to work this out. (28-year-old female, married 4 years)

With trepidation in her voice, this woman continued to explain that she was currently consulting with her attorney on ways to protect herself from physical violence in case she decided to end the marriage.

These responses illustrate the ambivalence and despair that accompanies thoughts of ending a marriage. It is a difficult decision to make, and disaffected spouses were expending a great deal of cognitive activity and emotional energy on making it.

Actions to End the Marriage

Unlike the previous phase in which respondents were thinking about ending their marriages but not acting on it, in this phase respondents were actually taking actions to dissolve their marriages. Whereas none of the respondents reported actions to dissolve the marriage in the beginning stage and 20% reported taking actions during the middle phase, 80% reported actions to end the marriage during the last phase. One third of the respondents at this stage had already physically separated. Many of the respondents reported ways in which they were trying to become more independent from their partner, for example, paying their own bills, not asking the partner for money, not depending on the partner for companionship.

> I'm getting a new job because I know I couldn't support myself and the baby on what I am making now. I've made calls about apartments, and I'm buying a second car. I've called about my insurance coverage and inquired about therapists. I've told more people. Before it was a major secret—I've told many more people. . . . I've told my family . . . that we haven't been getting along. I've thought about things like custody and visitation. (35-year-old female, married 5 years)

Although most of the disaffected spouses were taking actions to dissolve their marriages, 20% were not taking such actions. For these respondents, barriers—social, legal, financial, and emotional—stood in the way.

> I have an older sister and when we were home my parents always believed in "murder yes, divorce no." They were very strict against divorce. And although it was a standard joke with them—"murder yes, divorce no"—although my parents didn't show any real resentment when my sister divorced, I think down deep I was raised on that "murder yes, divorce no" issue and that it really hurt my parents when my sister got divorced. So, therefore, I was using our marriage to say, "I don't dare get divorced now because it would really double hurt them to know they've raised two failures." . . . We're sticking together because I don't want to hurt my parents. I've often thought that when my mother dies and I don't have any close relatives, I'll just walk out—I have nothing to lose then. That's a real possibility. . . . I'm not staying married because of my wife but because my family has put so much social pressure on that. (43-year-old male, married 21 years)

Final Efforts to Save the Marriage

As expected, during the end phase respondents spoke of fewer attempts to solve their marital problems. This was another indication that the respondents were moving away from repair toward dissolution. The disinterest in problem-solving attempts during the final phase parallels Ponzetti and Cate's (1986) finding that discussion of marital dissatisfactions was significantly less frequent during the last phase of the marital dissolution process. There may be no reason to discuss marital dissatisfactions if spouses are preparing to leave and have no investment in conflict resolution in the marriage at this point.

Disaffected spouses were more frequently turning to professional counselors for assistance during this phase. Until this stage, counseling was rarely pursued. But in the final phase 27% of the disaffected spouses were seeking counseling (compared to 12% during the middle phase). The last phase, then, was the most common time for marital therapy to be sought. But the reason for seeking counseling was not necessarily to repair the marriage. Often other motives were underlying the counseling, and the counseling was often initiated with a very pessimistic attitude toward saving the marriage.

> I'm not so sure I cared about the marriage counselor idea because I'm not that hot on it and I never was. . . . But I did mention it to him. And he said, okay. And I was really surprised that he said okay. Once he said okay, then I started wanting to go with him less and less. (32-year-old female, married 4 years)

> When we started counseling, the first time we came, I had had it in my mind that the marriage was going to end. I mean this was a last-ditch effort. I had already made it up in my mind that this marriage was not going to work and this was my last attempt. (26-year-old female, married 6 years)

Another respondent spoke of the ineffectiveness of counseling in helping her to cope with her marriage:

> At one point I tried to tell the pastor [about the marriage problems], but he just got the impression that the problems were just financial and that's how I got the job cleaning the church. He didn't understand that there were other problems. I tried to tell him, "I don't want my marriage to be ruined any more." . . . I was trying to explain to him that it was more than a financial problem. (28-year-old female, married 4 years)

Another respondent found the counseling personally helpful in coping with the marital problems. But since she was going alone to the counselor, she did not consider it effective in changing the marriage.

> I told myself things that I had learned or heard in counseling. . . . I saw other marriages with problems a lot worse where the people would work things out. But there were two people working together. This wound up to be so one-sided. I felt I had given it my all. . . .
>
> The counselor had told me, "You're only going to be able to handle this for so long. Some day it would reach a point when you won't be able to live with it." And that's kind of what happened. (43-year-old female, married 9 years)

Some respondents stated their reasons for not seeking professional help:

> He's never liked doctors or psychiatrists of any kind—very negative especially towards psychiatrists. I had no desire to seek marriage counseling either. Once I realized there was a problem in our relationship, I just wanted to end it—I really didn't care about seeing anyone. (32-year-old female, married 13 years)

> I was always afraid that a marriage counselor would want to for sure try to get us together and that they would find me at fault and that my husband would feel like I'm tattling on him. . . .

The way he is, he just isn't going to change. He just can't change. Maybe if he wanted to on his own get his therapy that way—maybe that would affect the marriage indirectly. He just doesn't seem like he would consider that. (32-year-old female, married 4 years)

Some respondents viewed a counselor as working only to repair the marriage and not to provide assistance in dissolving it. They feared that after all their contemplation and decision making about the marriage, they might be talked out of their decision to divorce or at least be unsupported by the counselor.

Other reasons, unrelated to repairing the marriage, were given for seeking counseling at this time.

I saw the psychiatrist—not to help him—but to make it look good in court records. I think more than anything, I didn't want his attorney to say, "Look, she's not even trying. The counseling would help him, and she's not doing that." (32-year-old female, married 13 years)

But I wanted to go to someone outside that didn't know us and see what they had to say. I don't think I went to counseling to work out the marriage because I really didn't think there was any hope for it. But I did want to see if they noticed the same thing in my husband that I did. (22-year-old female, married 4 years)

Again, social validation was important to the disaffected spouses. Receiving confirmation from an "expert" would give them further reassurance that they were doing the "right thing."

In general, passive and pleasing behaviors that were prevalent in the beginning and middle phases declined significantly in the end phase. The disaffected spouse's "pleasing" behaviors in earlier phases were an indirect way of trying to resolve problems, and these behaviors often stemmed from the disaffected spouse's feeling that he or she was responsible for the problems. During the last phase, most respondents were no longer blaming themselves for the problems nor feeling responsible for their solutions.

> I know that whatever actions he takes I'm not responsible for them. When we were younger and he would do something asinine, I always felt shame for it. Today I don't feel that way. I'm not responsible for his attitude or what comes out of his mouth. (46-year-old female, married 16 years)

Also, at this stage disaffected spouses no longer felt that they had to use indirect means to show their dissatisfaction to their partner. They could assert themselves in a very direct way because they had little to lose by doing so. During the initial phase of the disaffection process, the use of direct confrontation may have been too threatening or risky for relationship maintenance. Spouses will only reveal all of their dissatisfactions when "the costs of staying in the relationship are outweighed by the benefits of leaving" (Vaughan, 1986, p. 78). Hence, indirect behaviors such as passivity and attempts to please can be expected to occur less frequently during the end phase when the possibility of the dissolution of the marriage is considered more favorable.

Physical withdrawal was a very frequent behavior during the end phase—regardless of whether or not the spouses were choosing to dissolve the marriage. The reasons for withdrawal included (1) frustration over unsuccessful conflict resolution, (2) protection from further hurt, and (3) as an indirect way to get the partner's attention. But for some respondents, their withdrawal, which was psychological as well as physical, seemed to be a step toward dissolving the relationship.

The Partner's Reactions to Their Spouse's Disaffection

During the beginning phase of disaffection, the disaffected respondents had perceived few changes in their partner's behaviors, and any attempts by the partner to change were viewed by respondents as short-lived, token gestures of change. The respondents spoke of their partner's denial and a reluctance to admit marital problems. However, during the final phase, reports of partner denial declined significantly. Fewer than one half of those reporting partner denial in the beginning were reporting it at the end. In this final stage, the respondents were more assertive in expressing their discontent, making it difficult for their partner to continue to deny and ignore their marital problems. During this last phase it was more likely that respondents perceived their partner as attempting to repair the marriage. Apparently, the partners of the disaffected spouses still thought the marriage was salvageable, and they were making last-minute pleas to their spouse for another chance.

> When I decided to file, he said "I'll do anything." (23-year-old female, married 3 years)

> My husband came back to me and said he was very, very sorry. He really wanted a marriage with me. He had made a great mistake. Even if I couldn't forgive him, could I at least try to work on the marriage again. And I seriously considered it. I felt a lot of feelings of love for him; I had missed him a lot. We had so many fun things in common. It was a real dilemma for a full year to try to decide if I wanted him personally into my life and to work hard enough at our differences to make our marriage work. And only until the last month have I been able to say I don't feel in love—really, really feel in love. (30-year-old female, married 4 years)

> He was real supportive—worked tons of overtime so that I could go to graduate school. He did all the housework, he cooked, he did everything he could to help me get through school. (30-year-old female, married 11 years)

> He changed. He did all the things within reason that I wanted to do (for example, to go out). I thought he really had changed. We would go out, and he would sit there for a couple hours and we would talk. (42-year-old female, married 24 years)

When listening to the reported changes by the partners that occurred at this time, one wonders if the disaffection could have been prevented had these changes taken place at a much earlier time in the marriage. Before reaching the point of apathy and indifference, the partners' changes may have modified the respondents' perceptions of their partner and marriage, and subsequently restored positive feelings. The changes by the partners—even at this late stage—demonstrated that these partners were still quite invested in the relationship and, furthermore, that disaffection often occurs unilaterally. However, there were also cases of *mutual* disaffection. Several respondents reported that their partner was withdrawing and initiating separations.

> She spent a lot of time away from the house sorting out what she wanted. She was seeing another guy. (29-year-old male, married 6 years)

Lastly, some partners were perceived as defensive and denying that they had any problematic behaviors that contributed to the marital dissatisfaction.

> He responded with a lack of understanding and said, "You don't need your family." . . . He just couldn't understand my feelings. He couldn't understand the way I was brought up. He couldn't understand the closeness of my family. He thought that was very suffocating. I guess basically he couldn't comprehend anything different from the way he was brought up. He just doesn't realize that maybe his thinking is wrong, that he may be doing something wrong. (26-year-old female, married 6 years)

> My husband does not believe we have a problem in our marriage. And it almost makes me want to cry when I think about it. (28-year-old female, married 4 years)

> He thinks we're in the good days, and I'm thinking about how I'm going to leave. We're on different planets. And I feel bad

about how this is going to hit him. Because I know that in spite of me talking to him about therapy and everything else in the last 3 years, it's going to hit him like a ton of bricks. He acts out, and it really frightens me what he may do, and he doesn't have the resources in terms of support—family or friend support—that I have or even the internal resources to cope with it. (35-year-old female, married 5 years)

According to the respondents, some of the partners recognized the problems but still insisted that the disaffected respondent was the person with the problem. In the beginning of the disaffection process, the respondent probably shared this belief, but at the end they were less likely to believe that they were totally responsible for the problems.

He said, "You go to the counselor for a little while, and then maybe I'll go." Then every time we'd get into a fight he'd say, "Well, you go to your counselor, it's your problem. You're the one with the problem not me." (24-year-old female, married 4 years)

He stood beside me during my depression. When we talked to my psychiatrist, he told the psychiatrist that he was perfectly happy the way things had been—he was content. And I was throwing out all these things that I wasn't happy about anything. . . . He said he could only change so much. (54-year-old female, married 36 years)

He hasn't made any changes. He waits for me to calm down and see that he's right. (31-year-old female, married 2 years)

I express my concerns to her, but it's like yelling down a well. It seems like she lives in another world. When I would say something to her, she would just shrug it off or say, "Oh, you said that before." (38-year-old male, married 2 years)

The partners' defensive behaviors—denial, disagreeing, control, physical/verbal abuse—continued to contribute to the negative thoughts and feelings the respondents were already experiencing, and this discouraged the resolution of conflicts. Even when the disaffected spouses were trying to solve problems—either directly or indirectly—the partners resisted problem-solving attempts. These responses are typical of reciprocal negativity, which results when a spouse's complaint is not listened to but is met with a counterattack or withdrawal (Gottman, 1979). Thus, the disaffected spouse may return with a negative response or hold in anger and resentment, which accumulate over time.

Changes Desired by the Disaffected Spouses

It was apparent that the majority of respondents did not see their partner making changes, and those disaffected spouses who did see changes were not satisfied with them. To obtain a clearer picture of the kind of changes the respondents were looking for in their marriage, I asked them what changes needed to take place in order for them to feel better about their marriage. Eighty-eight percent of the respondents could think of changes they wanted (see Table 4.1 for a breakdown of desired changes). Twelve percent of the respondents stated that nothing would restore their feelings—it was too late.

> At this point I'm not sure that it can be saved. I'm not sure that there is anything either of us can do—short of me giving in and saying, "Okay I quit." I've reached the point where I don't really care. It's too late. As far as I'm concerned we did all this 5 years ago. I basically gave him a second chance 5 years ago—it lasted for a year or two. (42-year-old female, married 24 years)

Twenty percent of the respondents acknowledged that behavioral changes were actually taking place, but only one half of these respondents stated that these were resulting in any change in their feelings. Indeed, it appeared that for most of the respondents, any attempt to change by their partner was not going to rekindle their feelings of love.

TABLE 4.1 Changes Desired in the Marriage

	Percent[a]
Changes in partner's personality/attitude[b]	23
Partner discontinues control/domination	16
Partner engages in more intimate behaviors[c]	16
Couple develops ways to solve problems	12
Go to counseling (individual or marital)	7
Partner discontinues substance abuse	7
Partner shows more sexual interest	7
Respondent makes attitudinal changes[d]	5
Partner leaves	5
Partner discontinues contact with third party	2
	100

[a]Percentage of respondents ($N = 43$) who cited the change desired in the marriage.
[b]Admit problem and be motivated to work on marriage; strive for different type of marriage; make changes in values; have more self-confidence and trust.
[c]Behaviors such as empathy, understanding, companionship, and caring.
[d]Forget negative things from past; be less jealous of partner; be more open.

When the partner was finally willing to make changes, many of the disaffected spouses had reached a point of indifference, a point beyond which they no longer wanted to try to save the marriage. It was typically when the partner was ultimately faced with the possibility of divorce that he or she was more willing to try. But at this point the disaffected spouses felt that they had already tried—perhaps many times. The partner defined the relationship as salvageable, but the disaffected spouses did not. Consequently, when the couple sought marital therapy at this time, each spouse was likely to be approaching the therapy with different goals. For the disaffected spouses, the goal may have been to gain assistance in leave-taking or in insuring that the partner has a therapist to take care of him or her during an impending divorce. For the partner, often the goal was to repair the marriage.

If the partner did make behavioral changes, it was difficult for the disaffected spouses to acknowledge these changes if they had already made the decision to leave. The disaffected spouses could not allow themselves to feel a lot of hope and excitement about the partner's changes and be working on making a physical and psychological separation at the same time. One respondent stated that her husband wanted to do whatever it took to get back together. However, she had made her decision to leave, and although he was making changes, she didn't want to recognize them. She stated,

> I guess I was always trying to get him to do something to justify my leaving so that I would not feel the guilt when I did leave. (34-year-old female, married 12 years)

Likewise, this next respondent did not want to give the impression that if his wife changed, he would come back to her. Although she was trying to change, he had made up his mind about leaving.

> I don't have feelings of hate. I think that my wife is a fine person. It's just that we're two different people—in two different worlds. . . . There's apathy in that I don't let myself act in a positive way. . . . It may lull her into a false sense of security. (47-year-old male, married 20 years)

Vaughan (1986) observed a similar pattern among her subjects who were initiating marital dissolution.

> Initiators must appear to try and simultaneously convey the message that trying is not working. When the goal is separation, initiators cannot afford the luxury of sentiment. They can't make the break if they allow themselves to be moved by the partner's pleas, fears, attractiveness, or threats. If they are affected—even momentarily—they dare not show it, for the partner would take even the smallest signal as a possible change of heart. Initiators cultivate a stance toward the partner that is sufficiently angry or benevolent or detached to allow them to proceed toward physical separation, insulating themselves emotionally from the partner's efforts. (pp. 115–116)

The respondents choosing to end their marriages may have been trying to create an acceptable story for its ending. Indeed, a crucial part of coming to terms psychologically with the dissolution of a relationship is developing an account of the end of one's marriage (Duck, 1982). But when the partner is making positive changes, developing this account can be difficult to do unless one can ignore the positive changes made by the partner and continue to focus on the negative traits.

Coping with Disaffection

In general, the types of coping with marital disaffection changed from indirect and destructive behaviors to more direct and constructive coping strategies. For example, there were reductions in reports of silence, busyness, denial, and self-destructive behaviors. Toward the end of the disaffection process, spouses more frequently reported dealing directly with their problems through the use of professional help, confidants, and support groups (see Table 4.2). They were now involving family and friends to a greater degree as they began to disclose the marital dissatisfactions and elicit support from others. Until the disaffected spouses were serious about taking action to end the marriage, they were often reluctant to "go public" with their marital discontent.[1]

> I started to make more active coping. I called a friend . . . told her that I thought we were on the verge of splitting up. She offered her house for a short-term place to stay. (35-year-old female, married 5 years)

> Now I used my family. I moved in with them. This time I knew it was going to be permanent and that I would need the support. I definitely moved home. (24-year-old female, married 4 years)

> I just started to talk to my family since I decided to get a divorce. (30-year-old female, married 10 years)

TABLE 4.2 Coping Skills Utilized by Respondents during Marital Disaffection Process

Coping skill	Beginning percent[a]	End percent[b]
Confided in family or friend	43	57
Sought professional help	12	57***
Increased busyness	49	27*
Silence	53	12***
Avoidance	20	25
Denial	25	4**
Self-destructive behavior	18	2**
Increased involvement with family/friends	16	8
Joined support group	4	14
Attempts at own problem solving	8	2
Involvement with other sex	2	10
Spiritual practices	4	8
Talking/writing to self	10	2
Distanced psychologically	6	14

[a]Percentage of all respondents ($N = 49$) who cited this coping skill; total is more than 100% because of multiple responses.
[b]The asterisks indicate changes in coping according to the sign test.
*p <.05; **p <.01; ***p <.001.

I talked to my parents and friends—everyone of them are on my side. (24-year-old female, married 4 years)

I talked with a lot of friends and my mother. My friends stated that they didn't like my husband even before I had married him. (26-year-old female, married 6 years)

Gender differences in coping styles have been found in some studies on marital dissolution. Men have been found to use more denial and avoidance; women were more likely to turn to others for practical and/or emotional support or to accommodate by adapting themselves to the situation (Brown, 1976). Hagestad and Smyer (1982) also found that women sought social support during disengagement more frequently than men. In my study no clear-cut

gender differences were found on any of the coping styles. However, parallel to Brown's findings, there was a tendency for males to
more frequently report avoidance and for females to more often
report talking to a confidant and to be silent in the relationship (a
type of accommodation). Contrary to Brown's results, females in
my study tended to use denial just as often as males.

Summary

During this last phase, many loving feelings that once existed had
turned to apathy and indifference. While anger was still present,
hurt had decreased. In fact, several respondents stated they were
"beyond hurt." Pity for the partner was more common, but not
enough guilt was felt to keep many respondents from ending the
relationship. The loneliness experienced in earlier phases was being
alleviated through contacts with friends and family. The respondents were increasingly disclosing their marital disaffection to others.

Ending the marriage became a more predominant thought
during the final phase. And whereas in the previous phase it was
merely a thought, for many respondents in the end phase the
thought was being transformed into action as respondents took
specific steps to end their marriage. There continued to be a cognitive focus on the negative traits of the partner as some respondents prepared their personal accounts for leaving.

During this last phase problem-solving activities were fewer
since many respondents had given up hope that their partners
would change. Even in cases in which the partner made substantial
changes, the respondents described a "point of no return," that is,
a point beyond which feelings could no longer be restored. Unlike
previous phases, many disaffected spouses were pursuing professional counseling. Counseling was usually either a last desperate
effort to repair the marriage, or an arena in which to receive assistance for leave-taking, or a means by which to leave the partner in
good care.

Overview of the Marital Disaffection Process

Table 4.3 provides an overview of the phases of marital disaffection by listing the feelings, thoughts, and behaviors for each phase. This model of the disaffection process represents the process of disaffection that was most commonly followed by the respondents in my

TABLE 4.3 The Phases of Marital Disaffection

PHASE I: Disappointment

Feelings:	Anger, hurt, disillusionment
Thoughts:	Awareness of partner's flaws; thinking that marriage is not turning out as expected; assuming responsibility for relationship
Behaviors:	Attempts are made to solve marital problems unilaterally; person tries to please partner; avoidant and passive coping strategies (silence, denial) are used

PHASE II: Between Disappointment and Disaffection

Feelings:	Intense anger and hurt
Thoughts:	Partner's negative traits are viewed as a pattern; person evaluates the rewards and costs of marriage; person considers staying in marriage versus leaving it
Behaviors:	Person continues to attempt problem solving but more directly confronts partner about problems; person begins physical and emotional withdrawal from the marriage

PHASE III: Reaching Disaffection

Feelings:	Anger, apathy, hopelessness
Thoughts:	Making plans to end marriage; focus on partner's negative traits and attributing problems to partner; continued evaluation of rewards and costs of marriage
Behaviors:	Actions to dissolve marriage; attempts at problem solving; seeks counseling—usually to help disengage

study. Although there were some departures from this model, they were rare. The respondents differed on the actual time spent in each phase. Whereas some spouses went through all phases within a few years, others took as long as 25 years. An interesting area for further study would be to compare these two groups—the quick disaffectors and the slow-to-disaffect—on variables such as gender, age, coping, commitment, attractive alternatives, and so on.

In comparing the original model of the disaffection process proposed in Chapter 1 (see Table 1.1) with the model presented in Table 4.3, several differences are apparent. First, the original theoretical model consisted of five stages with distinct characteristics at each stage. The new model of the disaffection process contains three phases with some factors appearing in more than one phase. Phases II through IV (hurt, anger, and ambivalence) of the original model collapse into one middle phase in the new model. The feelings, thoughts, and behaviors of the three original phases occurred somewhat simultaneously in no particular sequence or ordering. Second, the feeling of ambivalence is notably absent from any of the phases of the disaffection process in the new model. Respondents rarely reported this feeling and, hence, it did not appear as a primary feeling during any of the phases. Although they did not report feeling ambivalent, their thoughts of evaluating the rewards and costs of the marriage and deciding whether to stay or leave are an indication of some ambivalence. Third, in the new model there was a tendency for the disaffected spouses to assert marital dissatisfaction to the partner early in the process rather than later, as originally proposed. Fourth, anger and awareness of the partner's negative traits appeared in the new model in the beginning phase, whereas based on the original model they were expected to occur in the middle of the process.

Note

1. For a few respondents, participating in my research study was "going public" with their disaffection for the first time, since they had not told

anyone else about their disaffection. In fact, it appeared that some of the respondents participated in the study in order to have someone listen to and validate their feelings, or even to get assistance in making a decision. (It was clearly stated in the consent form that therapy was not a part of the interview.)

What Causes Love to Die?

We just grew apart and we had different ideas about how mar-
riage should be and what a relationship should be.
(24-year-old female, married 4 years)

Most spouses experience some dissatisfactions or marital doubts
during the course of their marriages. However, they all do not fall
out of love. What drives some marriages then to continue down the
road of disaffection while others can survive the marital bumps and
maintain love? There is no singular reason for love to die, but
several overarching themes were apparent in the interviews. In this
chapter the major reasons for the disaffection as reported by the
respondents will be examined. In addition, we will look at some of
the driving forces that pushed the spouses to move from one phase
to the next.

Mutuality and Control

A majority of the respondents claimed that there was a lack of
mutuality in their marital relationship. Mutuality is a respectfulness
for one another based on the belief that each individual is an equal
partner in the relationship. Any act that involves controlling or
dominating a partner, or disregards consideration of a partner's
opinions, desires, activities, and life-style, or that forces a spouse to
do something against his or her will demonstrates a lack of mutuality. Behaviors that indicate lack of mutuality are criticizing, in-

ability to compromise, attempts to alienate friends of the spouse, jealous behaviors, and psychological/emotional smothering. For the most part, the behaviors described by respondents were not violent or physically abusive, but they were emotionally abusive. Napier (1988) refers to the lack of mutuality in relationships as "interpersonal inequity," which he defines as the "imbalance in vital determination of whose experience, whose feelings, had most importance" (p. 78). The marriage with interpersonal inequity usually consists of a narcissistic partner—the emotional "taker"—and a self-denying partner—the emotional "giver."

More than one half of the respondents (53%) cited as turning points in their marriages a partner's attempt to control them. Typical examples of a partner's controlling behavior were situations in which a decision was made unilaterally by the partner, disregarding the disaffected respondent's opinion. Examples of such decisions were how the respondent should dress, where they should live, how they should spend money, and so on. Some of them were major life decisions—others were quite minor. But the common element was the lack of consideration for the respondent's input, opinions, and feelings in the decision-making process.

After the respondents recounted their process of disaffection, I asked them what contributed most to their dissatisfaction about their relationship? My hope was to elicit the overall cause of their disaffection. One of the two most frequent responses was the partner's controlling behavior (see Table 5.1). The following quotes typify this response:

> His bullying of me—that I couldn't disagree with him verbally even in a very controlled way without his getting furious. That I have to be very passive and pretend to agree with him and go along with what he says. He thinks we have a very egalitarian marriage. But it doesn't feel that way to me. (35-year-old female, married 5 years)

> If he would let me have some expression of my own. For example, in decorating the house—he won't let me do any-

TABLE 5.1 "What Contributes *Most* to Your Dissatisfaction With Your Relationship?"

	Percent[a]
1. Partner's control	20
2. Partner's lack of intimate behaviors	20
3. Partner's other negative trait (e.g., disloyalty, overdependence, inability to give, etc.)	14
4. Partner's inability to resolve problems	8
5. Different life-styles	8
6. Partner's lack of sexual interest	6
7. Partner's passivity	6
8. Different marital expectations	4
9. Partner's substance abuse	4
10. Confrontations with in-laws	2
11. Partner's lack of financial support	2
12. Respondent's self-esteem	2
13. Unfulfilled expectations	2
	98[b]

[a]Percentage of respondents ($N = 49$) who cited this factor as among those that contribute to their overall marital dissatisfaction.
[b]Total is due to rounding off percentages.

thing. If he would just let me go ahead and fix the home. (56-year-old female, married 25 years)

His complete lack of feeling for my feelings. You cannot look at him and say, "Please don't do that because it really hurts me and this is why." He will just say, "Well if it hurts you and bothers you that's your problem. Because I'm just going to keep on doing it." That's how he is. So that's why it's so hard to be with him. It's either be exactly the way he wants you to be or don't be with him. (31-year-old female, married 2 years)

This last response, in particular, portrays the absence of a critical component of mutuality—empathy. Mutual empathy conveys an understanding and acceptance of the feelings of the partner—even feelings that are different from one's own.

> Mutual empathy occurs when two people relate to each other in a context of interest in the other, emotional availability and responsiveness, cognitive appreciation of the wholeness of the other; the intent is to understand. While some mutual empathy involves an acknowledgment of the sameness in the other, an appreciation of the differentness of the other's experience is also vital. The movement toward the other's differentness is actually central to growth in relationships and also can provide a powerful sense of validation for both self and other. (Jordan, 1991, p. 89)

Not only does mutual empathy validate a spouse's self-concept but it encourages the *development* of the self-concept. Jordan (1991) explains, "Through empathy, and an active interest in the other as a different, complex person, one develops the capacity at first to allow the other's differentness and ultimately to value and encourage those qualities that make that person different and unique" (p. 82). Without mutual empathy and acknowledgement of the other's feelings by the partner, the spouses may view their feelings and ideas as invalid or illegitimate. One disaffected wife described the effects of her husband's nonacceptance of her feelings with the following:

> I think the loss of my identity as a human being, as a person having comments or anything that were of any value and being able to contribute something—nothing was of value. (43-year-old female, married 9 years)

A controlling partner who has no desire for a mutual relationship but only a relationship that serves his or her needs will not care about their spouse's feelings. The partner fears his or her spouse's different feelings and ideas because the differentness is perceived as interfering with what the partner wants. By discounting, ignoring, or minimizing the spouse's feelings and desires, the controlling partner can proceed with what he or she wants to do. Unfortunately, in the process, the spouse does not feel the "powerful sense of validation" that derives from mutual empathy. Rather than self-enhancement, low self-esteem, feelings of hurt and rejection, and resentment toward the controlling partner develop. Marriages in which partners engage in high level of criticism or coercion are almost universally unhappy (Napier, 1988).

When respondents were asked what changes needed to take place in order for them to feel better about the marriage, the following responses again reflect the desire for mutuality in the marriage:

> He would have to stop wanting to be the dominant one—the boss, the leader. He would have to be much more sensitive to all feelings, and not just his. (31-year-old female, married 2 years)

> I would like for him to be more open and for a relationship like women have with close girlfriends, being able to talk with that person with no judgement cast down on you—a give-and-take relationship. (26-year-old female, married 8 years)

While a controlling and domineering partner was cited by both women and men as a reason for falling out of love, women and men differed on their expectations for power. Women's complaints about their husbands' control emerged from their desire for an equitable relationship. When first married, many of the women adhered to traditional gender roles that prescribed the husband to be the head of the household. This was especially true for those women who married during the 1950s, when this was the social norm for marriages. However, over the past three decades expectations for marriage have changed such that many women want to develop equal partner marriages, and they resent the traditional arrangement of male dominance.

> I had the realization that when we got married I was helpless and very dependent. He was a take-charge person, and I

wanted somebody who would take care of me and make all the decisions, and that's what I wanted. That's what he wanted to do—someone he could take care of and make all the decisions and have control over. That was fine with me—that was fine for both of us. But then I realized that I had grown, and I was no longer helpless and dependent, and I didn't want this anymore. So I blamed that—the fact that I had changed and that he was trying to resist this change, even though he thought that's what he wanted. He didn't want someone lying on the couch unable to get up for dinner, but he still didn't want someone he couldn't control. So I blamed it on that—the fact that there was this change going on. (53-year-old female, married 21 years)

Interestingly, one respondent who complained about her husband's control also expressed some ambivalence in his relinquishing it.

I had agoraphobia, and if I got better I would be more independent. And he liked me being dependent on him. He said his mother was that way—dependent on his dad. . . . My husband reminds me of dad, who was so domineering all the time. . . .

The problem is I want my independence in some ways but truthfully in other ways I don't. With my agoraphobia, to me it's a much easier life with not being independent, in other words, having him drive me places and stuff like that. (28-year-old female, married 4 years)

When the disaffected husbands complained about their wife's power or control, it was because they expected to be the dominant spouse, and it was not turning out that way. Notice how the following male respondents complained about their wife's assertiveness as a challenge to their authority.

I had expected her to stay at home . . . to give up everything for me. She came from a conservative family and although she had earned a master's degree, I thought she would give up her career for me. (68-year-old male, married 36 years)

She wanted to do it her way and didn't see anything wrong with it. . . . I just felt like I was there to be a plumber or repairman. I'd cut the grass, fix the pipes. As far as being a father or a head of the household, I wasn't. (49-year-old male, married 26 years)

Whereas both men and women in this sample voiced complaints about a controlling partner, for men it was seen as a threat to their authority and for women as a threat to an equitable relationship. This was especially true for a subgroup of older men in the sample who still adhered to the traditional gender roles in marriage.

Even when spouses want to develop equal partner marriages, this is not easily transformed into actual behavior changes. Many men are apparently still behaving according to the norm in which the husband maintains a dominant position in the marriage (and their wives behave accordingly), even though men and women may profess contrary views.

> Because male-female relationships are so laden with stereotyped expectations, particularly around dominance and submission, it is often difficult to establish mutuality even though both partners deeply long for it. Often mutuality comes more easily for women in woman-to-woman relationships, which can provide wonderfully sustaining mutual empathy and care. (Jordan, 1991, p. 89)

Thus, sex role norms (particularly for men) have not altered to align themselves to changing marital expectations of being equal partners. Unfortunately, a consequence of this imbalance of power is that the subordinate person feels devalued and not respected as a mature adult. A self-enhancing relationship for *both* partners evolves only through interdependence, equality, and mutual respect. A relationship of mutuality enhances both spouses' sense of competence, of acceptance, and of being valued. A sense of mutuality conveys "an appreciation of the wholeness of the other person with a special awareness of the other's subjective experience" (Jordan, 1991, p. 82).

Lack of Emotional Intimacy

Partner's lack of emotional intimacy shared top ranking with partner's control as the major contributor to marital dissatisfaction (see Table 5.1). Respondents described their dissatisfactions with the level of intimacy in a variety of ways. They talked about "missing romance," "the lack of togetherness in the sense of doing things together," "emotional nonsupport," "inability to understand my feelings," "problems with being intimate and sharing," "lack of companionship," and "lack of emotional attachment." The aspects of intimacy that respondents most commonly reported were missing from their marriages included self-disclosure, emotional support, and companionship. One respondent vividly described her dissatisfaction with the level of intimacy in her marriage with the following:

> He wasn't intimate. . . . That is something I need—I need to have someone that I can share time with—all of me—my thoughts, feelings, everything. He just stopped doing that, and the whole marriage got mechanical. He wanted his physical needs to be met—feeding him, sex, take care of him and wash his clothes—just all of that. And there was no more romance, and I think that has to be there—at least a little bit. And just the communication—there wasn't any—everything was taken for granted with him. This is the way we do it, and there's no need to talk about it. And there was no privacy—there was always time with his family. (31-year-old female, married 3 years)

Frequent dissatisfaction with the level of emotional closeness further demonstrates the importance of the expressive aspects of marriage. The disaffected spouses wanted a marital relationship in which they could share their innermost feelings, with the accompanying acceptance of these feelings by their partner. They wanted a relationship in which love came unconditionally. Instead what they experienced was alienation and loneliness with a partner who was emotionally "miles away." What then prevented these spouses from attaining emotional closeness in their marriages?

As described in the previous section, part of the problem may be the controlling behavior of the partner. Spouses do not feel safe in expressing their private feelings and being open when a partner controls, dominates, and bosses them. Hence, intimacy cannot thrive in a relationship in which a partner intimidates by criticizing and belittling the spouse's opinions and feelings, not allowing free expression of ideas. Intimidation and control convey nonacceptance and devaluation of the other person.

Another reason for the lack of intimacy in some of the relationships was substance abuse. Approximately one third of the respondents stated that their partner's substance abuse affected their feelings toward their partner. The capacity for trust and self-esteem—prerequisites for the development of intimacy—are often impaired in a substance abuser. Drug abusers and alcoholics are often fearful of intimacy, making spouses in substance abuse systems struggle around closeness and distance in their interaction. Once the substance is eliminated from the family environment and many of the issues specific to their interaction around the substance abuse have been addressed, the couples can work at establishing greater intimacy (Bepko & Krestan, 1985).

Although many of the disaffected spouses reported that they had withdrawn sexually from their partner during the course of their disaffection, only three respondents reported that the lack of sexual intimacy contributed to their overall marital dissatisfaction. Apparently the sexual withdrawal was more symptomatic of the lack of their loving feelings, as opposed to it producing their disaffection in the first place.

Ineffective Conflict Resolution

The inability to resolve conflicts was a major contributor to the growing disaffection of the respondents throughout the disaffection process. Repeated failed attempts at problem solving by the dis-affected spouse were quite common. Typically, the difficulty in solving problems revolved around ineffective communication—poor speaking *and* listening skills by both the respondent and partner.

> We tried to talk, but he's not a very good talker. It seemed like I did most of the talking. And it would just go in one ear and out the other, so I quit talking. Then sometimes I was yelling—trying to yell it into his brain, I guess. That didn't work. (26-year-old female, married 8 years)

> I could talk to him until I was blue in the face, but he didn't listen. He didn't absorb what I was saying. I couldn't make him understand what I was saying. (42-year-old female, married 24 years)

Sometimes the problem was the *lack* of communication:

> I never discussed it or brought it up to her—Well, maybe in the heat of an argument, maybe something was said. One of the problems was that my wife and I could not sit and discuss anything—really totally talk about it. (47-year-old male, married 25 years)

> We never talked about it. But he could tell by my actions I wasn't liking it. I could tell he was very disappointed in me too. But there was nothing I could do about it; I didn't feel good. (54-year-old female, married 36 years)

Withdrawal was often a strategy taken by one of the partners during a conflict. Needless to say, withdrawing during conflict only led to further frustration and ineffective resolution as it was often interpreted as a punitive action by the one who was left behind.

> The more assertive I got, the more angry and sullen he would get. Sort of, "You don't want me anymore. You're picking on

me." Immature behavior. He would withdraw, he wouldn't talk, instead he would sulk. (32-year-old female, married 13 years)

I would try to confront her with my perceptions and feelings of the situation . . . It's highly unsuccessful because she tends to take my feelings differently and that I'm telling her that her feelings are wrong. I try to assure her that her feelings are not wrong. . . . We go through the same process over and over, and then eventually I go through a withdrawal process. (39-year-old male, married 17 years)

Another obstacle to conflict resolution was the partner's reluctance to compromise:

I didn't have any intentions of leaving. Somewhere along the line we would have to come to some type of an agreement. Somewhere there he was going to give in on something where we would be able to work and go on from there and keep the marriage together. I didn't have any desire get a divorce. (43-year-old female, married 9 years)

Finally, negative reciprocity impeded successful resolution of conflicts:

During our fights my wife would be very vindictive and I would sometimes retaliate. Once when she broke my records, I took a file and scratched her albums. I just wanted to make her realize what she was doing because I don't think she realized the basis of what she was doing. I've always tried to reason with her, but it doesn't seem to work. (38-year-old male, married 2 years)

Lacking a satisfactory way to resolve differences and dissatisfactions is very serious and can lead a spouse to leave a marriage—first emotionally, then possibly physically (Hite, 1987). Unresolved conflicts and inadequate behavior changes contribute to the continuing accumulation of hurts and increased anger. Although there is a paucity of research examining the association of the level of love with conflict resolution abilities, it is quite clear that inadequate conflict resolution does play a role in distressed marriages (Gottman, 1979; Raush, Barry, Hertel, & Swain, 1974). An accumulating effect of inadequate conflict resolution for married couples can occur as "every conflict and every resolution, as well as every failure at resolution, become part of the history whose effects determine the occurrence and course of further conflicts" (Peterson, 1983, p. 363).

Another problematic way of handling conflict in marriage is avoidance: Unresolved issues are never brought up. Partners who use the avoidance pattern become increasingly separate from one another in order to avoid confrontations, thereby gradually breaking off most interactions and connections to each other (Levinger, 1983). While avoidance may promote a peaceful coexistence, the interpersonal problems can increase, and disaffection then grows.

Shift in Attributions for Problems

For the most part, we have been examining behaviors of disaffected spouses and their partners that encouraged the development of disaffection in marriage. Underlying these overt types of actions were the more covert processes of the disaffected spouses' thinking. A shift in attributions for marital problems is a cognitive process that influenced the progression of disaffection. An attribution is a person's cognitive explanation of human behavior. In this study, attributions were categorized into four types: (1) *extradyadic*—events and people outside of the couple, for example, "death of friend," "child's illness," "financial problems"; (2) *partner*—characteristics of the partner, for example, "my spouse's selfishness," "my spouse's aggressiveness; (3) *self*—characteristics of the self, for example, "my own selfishness," "my own lack of self-disclosure"; and (4) *interactive*—features of the dyadic unit itself, for example, "we could not communicate," "the way my spouse and I solve disagreements."

Very few studies on attributions analyze attributions as an ongoing process. One exception to this is a study by Stephen (1987) on relationship termination. He explored the possibility that as time passed there would be a shift in the attribution of responsibility for the ending of an intimate relationship. In his study, a longitudinal design was used to follow changes in the couples' relationships over time, including the breakup process for couples who split up. The subjects who broke up were individually administered breakup questionnaires. Stephen (1987) found a positive association between the use of interpersonal (or interactive) attributions and positive coping with relationship termination for all subjects; but this association was stronger for females than males. Also, for females, the longer the amount of time between the terminating event and the administration of the questionnaire, the more frequently interpersonal and external attributions were used. This finding indicates that for females, there is a possible decrease in anger toward the partner with time since the partner is no longer totally blamed for marital problems.

In the present study, respondents reported using all four types of attributions throughout all the phases of disaffection. However, there was a significant decrease in self and extradyadic attributions over time (see Figure 5.1). Thus, partner attributions became more salient attributions during the end phase of disaffection as the other two types of attributions became less frequent.

Why were self and extradyadic attributions more common in the beginning phase of disaffection? Initially these attributions may be used to preserve the idealistic image of the partner—the "distortion" that Berger and Roloff (1982) have presented (see Chapter 2, this volume). This idealization of the partner is important to maintain since one does not want to admit that one has made a poor choice of a marriage partner. In a sense, it is also easier to maintain this positive perception of the partner since there has not yet been a history of hurts, anger, and negative thoughts about the person. After experiencing extensive hurts and offenses by the partner, a spouse is more inclined to blame the partner for marital problems.

The frequent use of extradyadic attributions during the begin-

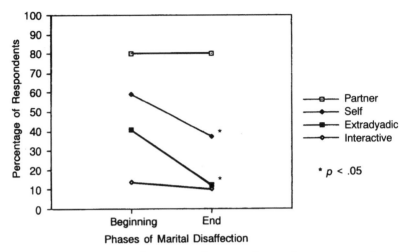

FIGURE 5.1 Respondents' attributions during beginning and end phases of marital disaffection.

ning phase of disaffection may be one reason respondents did not take assertive and direct actions to deal with their marital problems when they were first emerging. By attributing problems to extradyadic factors, the causes of the problems are perceived as being both out of one's control and not the responsibility of the partner. Therefore, directly confronting the partner is not viewed as a particularly effective action to take since the responsibility lies primarily with the extradyadic factor. For example, confronting the partner about financial problems in the marriage may make sense if the problems are perceived as stemming from the partner's overspending. But confronting the partner may be an inappropriate action if the spouse is blaming external factors, such as the poor economy and the cost of the children's college tuition, for the financial stress in the marriage.

During the beginning phase of disaffection the explanations for the marital problems were often quite complex, and respondents did not identify one specific type of attribution. The following statement illustrates the complexity of a respondent's explanation for a problem that she was experiencing early in the marriage.

He never had any children, he was almost 30 and used to living a certain way, and all of a sudden he's married and had two kids. So he was frustrated because things weren't working the way he thought they should work, and he's a really strict controlling person anyway, and I understood that, and that's why I was more patient with it than some other people. . . .

I did think that I was responsible too. He would say that I didn't take care of them right, so he had to do that. I didn't discipline them, so he had to do that. At first I accepted that and then I realized that no, maybe he's wrong. Maybe he expects too much from these children and from me. . . . Yeah, at first I just took what he was saying and thought maybe he is right and my kids are too unruly. But it changed. . . . I was willing to work it out with him. We really needed to work together. But no, he wanted it all. He felt that he was the man, so he had to control everything.

He has a family that's big, and they all stick together and take care of each other. . . . His sister would tell me, "Well, you just have to submit. He's the head of the house. And you have to do what he says. And you're not letting him be the head." And I think she was talking to him. . . . I felt like I had married the *whole* family, and I had to change all of my ways in order to suit them. (31-year-old female, married 3 years)

This account contains attributions that include: (1) extradyadic factors (her children, her in-laws), (2) the partner (his inexperience with children, his controlling personality), (3) the self ("I was responsible too"), and (4) interactive factors (their inability to work together to resolve differences in child rearing).

At the end of the disaffection process, the attributional accounts were less complex and more unidimensional. They seemed to focus on one or, at most, two causes. At this stage, the partner attribution was the one most frequently used. The increase in partner attributions may partly be explained by the fact that a greater number of respondents were actually ending their relationships during this phase. They may have felt compelled to arrive at a face-saving explanation for the dissolution of the marriage. During the last stage of relationship disengagement, the person's "accounts may reflect bias, idealization, self-interest," but they play a psychologically critical role in dealing with the relationship dissolution (Duck, 1982). By blaming the partner, the person can justify his or her action to dissolve the marriage and thus alleviate at least some degree of guilt. In a similar vein, some research suggests that among those individuals asking for a divorce, attributions toward one's partner may be used as a means to distance oneself from the partner (Newman & Langer, 1981).

Many of the accounts of the process of disaffection revealed the shift from blaming oneself or extradyadic factors to a total blaming of the partner. For a 43-year-old female respondent who had been married 9 years, her disaffection began during the second year of her marriage when her husband displayed an unreasonable and uncaring attitude toward her children from a previous marriage. When asked what accounted for the problems, she attributed the problems to herself and her inability to have children with him. She stated:

> There must be something where I'm coming up short on what I'm doing. But I didn't know what it was. I think to some degree he resented the fact that we couldn't have children, especially when something went wrong with my son or daughter. He may have felt that if we had one of our own, that wouldn't be happening—the same kind of problem going on—that he could have controlled it maybe with his own child.

During the middle phase of her disaffection process, this respondent was still taking total responsibility for the marital problems they were experiencing.

> I just didn't want to see that he couldn't change. I felt there must be some power within me that somehow there must be something that I could do to change him—that he cared

enough for me—that there was something I could say that would get us back.

By the end of the disaffection process, she had shifted the responsibility for their problems onto her husband. When asked what accounted for her current marital problems, she stated:

> His [her husband's] personality. Maybe I contributed to it in some way—and I'm sure I did—but not to the extreme that it was. I think if he had given in a little on some things, I think we would have been able to make it. I was willing to accept so much of the blame. If he had accepted a little bit of it, I probably would have stayed.

A 30-year-old respondent, married 4 years, started the disaffection process with blaming herself for the marital problems. When there was disagreement with her husband over her clothes, she placed the responsibility on herself.

> I'm at fault. I accept all blame. I accept all fault. I don't like the boat rocked and accepting the blame is the easiest way not to rock it.

By the middle phase of her disaffection, she was still blaming herself. She attributed an argument in which he disapproved of her job to the following:

> There was a sense there that I had brought it back on myself. You can do something if you make it your responsibility. And because he did come up with some very logical arguments for these things, I thought, "maybe my perception is wrong."

However, by the end of the disaffection process, she was putting the responsibility for the marital problems on her husband.

> I feel that he'll never change. I think it would take a major,

major trauma in his life. Now I think he has a real serious problem, and I feel sorry for him as a human being and that he needs some help.

It is interesting to note the connection between attributions and the hope for change in the marriage. As long as the disaffected spouses felt responsible for the problems, they were hopeful for change. When the responsibility for problems was placed on the partner, their hope dwindled. Their feelings toward their partner were now totally dependent on their partner making changes—an unlikely prospect for many of them. Hence, a sense of hopelessness ensues when blame is totally placed on the partner.

Another change in the attributional activity of spouses that occurs during the process of disaffection is the increasing rigidity and inflexibility of the partner attributions. When there is a history of marital conflict and an escalation of conflict, over time a process develops whereby an individual's blame-oriented causal attributions rigidify (Howe, 1987). Furthermore, these rigid attributions can contribute to the negative emotions felt by the spouse by increasing his or her sensitivity to the negative actions of the partner. Blaming the partner may lead to negative exchanges that reinforce the blame-oriented beliefs of the spouse and consequently deepen the conflict cycle (Howe, 1987). The anger and frustration that accompanies the blaming of the partner may actually reduce a person's ability to see problems from an interactive or dyadic perspective (Howe, 1987).

An interactive attribution requires a more complex view of the situation, and when people are reacting with intense anger or hurt, they are likely to resort to a single, simple view of the cause of the problem. But if they are able to look at the problem from an interactive perspective, less volatile and extreme emotions are experienced. Take as an example the following fictitious case of a wife's attributional thinking:

Jane is not looking forward to her in-laws' visit this summer. Every summer during their 5-year marriage, Ned's parents and younger brother have visited for 2 weeks. Jane would prefer that she and her husband travel somewhere alone during their summer vacation instead of entertaining her in-laws. As the date of their arrival approaches, she begins to feel the strain and tension in Ned's and her marriage. In trying to explain what accounts for the problem, Jane has a couple of alternatives. First, she can blame Ned and attribute the problem to his inconsideration of her needs and his inability to stand up to his parents. She can dwell on how he does not understand her desires and lacks empathy for her feelings. If she chooses this line of attributional thinking, she will likely become more frustrated with and angrier at Ned as she anticipates her in-laws' arrival. Depending on how she handles her anger, it may potentially create additional negative feelings and actions between Ned and her.

A second alternative for Jane is to attribute the marital tension to the inability of Ned and her to openly discuss the decision to invite his family for their summer vacation. She thinks that this situation is typical of many decisions in their relationship in which each partner assumes what the other one wants without checking it out. Jane fears that if she doesn't assert herself and decisions are not discussed between them, the pattern will continue. Jane hopes that Ned will be understanding of her feelings when she discloses them to him and that this will lead to better problem solving when future conflicts arise.

Note the difference in the emotional overtone. The partner attributions elicit frustration and anger. The interactive attributions, however, provide a sense of hope and encouragement about the potential resolution of the problem. By taking mutual responsibility for the problem, spouses can be more hopeful that they can make changes in their relationship. When blame is cast on only one partner, it becomes a matter of trying to force the other person to change. And, as mentioned previously, the continual focus on the other's faults can produce an exaggerated picture of that person's flaws, which further reinforces the idea that the partner is to be blamed.

Hence, when marital problems are no longer being attributed to oneself, extradyadic events, or dyadic interactions, the source of problems narrows down to the partner. The partner attributions then play a significant role in the evolution of disaffection: The continual blaming of the partner for marital problems creates increasingly negative feelings toward the partner, and ultimately, if this process is not stopped, disaffection occurs.

Individual Happiness Becomes a Higher Priority

A successful marriage does not mean that spouses always place the partner's needs and happiness before their own. However, many people are socialized in traditional and religious values that prescribe selflessness as a necessary requirement for a successful marriage. But continual self-denial over time can rob a person of fulfillment of his or her own needs and ultimately change one's feelings about the marital relationship.

> I was raised by Christian missionaries. And we were always taught J-O-Y. Jesus first, then Others, Yourself always comes last. Unfortunately that was so ingrained in me that I practiced it. I'm sure that was part of the problem in the marriage. He always had to come first. (30-year-old female, married 4 years)

Behaving throughout the marriage as if one's own needs are not important and continually accommodating to the other person result in growing resentment, bitterness, and ultimately, disaffection. Upon realizing this, spouses may attempt to communicate to their partner the importance of their happiness. But when the style of the marriage has already become a rigid, long-standing pattern of the spouse serving the needs of the partner, it may be difficult to change.

As long as the disaffected spouses were more concerned about their partner's happiness (and/or, in many cases, their children's happiness) than their own, they felt obligated to stay in the marriage. Until they could begin to consider the importance of their own needs and desires, they were unaware of inequities in the relationship. For many, by putting their own happiness first, they were able to think seriously about their disaffection and, for some spouses, the possibility of leaving the relationship. Therefore, in order for a spouse to end the marital relationship, there needed to be a dramatic shift from commitment to others to commitment to self. Taking responsibility for one's own happiness became a priority.

> I have always felt sorry for everybody and now I'm thinking, "What about myself?" I've always put everybody from 1 to 20 and I was 20. And now all of a sudden I want to be 1—I want to do what's good for me for a change. (54-year-old female, married 36 years)

If the relationship no longer contributed to the disaffected spouse's personal growth, and personal growth was regarded as important, he or she felt justified in terminating it.

While maintaining the marriage for other people's happiness may be a noble and selfless gesture, some respondents discovered that it was not a particularly good reason for staying in a devitalized marriage. One husband, married for 25 years, described his experience with this motivation:

> I should never have stayed in the marriage this long. I should have gotten out when I knew that it wasn't going to work. Staying in may have been the best thing for other people, but it sure wasn't the best thing for me. (57-year-old male, married 25 years)

Another women decided it was not too late to get out, and she also thought that maintaining the marriage solely for her husband's happiness was not a good reason for staying.

> I've been so overridden by him that I've denied a large part of myself for these several years. And so leaving him and being on my own is the way to get myself back, and now I think it's the *only* way to get myself back. I think it would take major work on his part to allow me to be myself when that means being different from him. I don't see that happening—maybe I'm not being optimistic enough, but he's a very unhappy person,

and I think I married him because I thought I would be the one
to make him happy. I think I'm angry at him for not responding to my care. . . . I'm getting to the point where it's time to
throw in the towel on him. (35-year-old women, married 5
years)

Note the transition from self-denial to a desire for asserting her
own identity and individuality. Many of these respondents were
searching for validation and some attention to their own needs from
their partner. This emerging awareness of the legitimacy of their
own needs and happiness played a powerful role in the process of
disaffection. It compelled them to expect more from their relationship. And when fulfillment was not forthcoming, they began to
evaluate and scrutinize more closely their partner and the marital
relationship.

Alternative Attractions

The process of marital disaffection does not occur in a social vac-
uum. What is happening in the person's environment may also be
contributing to his or her feelings toward the partner. Each individual, whether consciously or not, is cognizant of possible alternatives outside the marriage (Thibaut & Kelley, 1959). Hence,
another driving force in the process of disaffection is the awareness
of alternative attractions. When spouses are no longer attracted to
their partner, they begin to look outside the marriage for the love
and attention lacking in their marriage. By finding attractions outside the marriage, what is left inside the marriage often appears pale
in comparison. When disaffected spouses discover that there are
better choices for a partner (whether in fantasy or reality) or that
there are other goals to pursue (e.g., getting a degree or job), they
become even less emotionally invested in their current relationship.
Therefore, even if the disaffected spouses in my study were not
terminating their marriage, they were likely to be investing less
in it.

The alternative to the marriage was not necessarily another

person. Basically, the individual expected a more pleasant existence outside the marital bond, whether in a new interpersonal relationship or in living alone. For some, the attraction was pursuing activities that had been put aside while investing time in the marriage. When asked what alternatives to the marriage were being pursued, respondents cited a variety of them, including the following:

> Since I've retired there are not enough hours in the day to do the things I enjoy doing. . . . I started a water exercise class . . . I go five mornings a week. I've just started also going to the Senior Citizens' exercise class. . . . I've signed up for tennis lessons. I do volunteer work at the hospital. I'm doing a good job there, and they appreciate me. All the other things I do [in the marriage] are not appreciated. I'm filling my life up with other things. (57-year-old female, married 33 years)

> What I'm putting my energy into is my kids, which is mostly what I was putting my energy in before. But at least I had him to be there with one kid while I'm chauffeuring the other kid. . . . Physically I'm spending more time with them. . . . Once I get a divorce, I'll have to do something about a job. (53-year-old female, married 21 years)

> For the first time this past year I have caught myself being attracted and interested in other men. I've met someone. . . . When I go out, I take off my wedding ring. If I met anyone, I was going to tell him I wasn't married. But I met this man, I guess I'm too honest. I couldn't lie.
>
> I'm keeping myself going as many hours in the day. (42-year-old female, married 24 years)

> At first I met somebody and that looked fairly promising—I went out with her for about two months. It was very much a friendship type of thing. Dating but not anything serious. I met this one girl who wants a relationship, and she's very quick to move into this. I'm not ready for this thing at all.

I'm trying to make friends to alleviate the loneliness. I have a roommate who moved into the house about a month ago. (30-year-old male, married 7 years)

Alternative attractions were most frequently mentioned during the last phase of marital disaffection. This is consistent with R. Miller (1982), another study on marital breakups, which found that attractions outside the marriage were reported by the majority of ex-spouses during the last phase of the process of marital breakdown.

The increase in the pursuit of alternative attractions is consistent with the decrease in loneliness during the last phase. Respondents reported more loneliness during the beginning and middle phases of disaffection when they were still highly invested in the marriage and concentrating their efforts on making the marriage work. Pursuing alternatives to the marriage during the end phase alleviated some of this loneliness through involvement in other interpersonal relationships and activities. Not all respondents were pursuing alternatives because they were ending their marriage. Many of them were getting involved in new relationships and activities in order to supplement the marriage and to cope with the emotional and social emptiness they felt within the marital relationship.

Summary

The three factors most frequently cited by respondents as causes of their disaffection related to difficulties in the interaction between spouses, namely, lack of mutuality, unfulfilled intimacy needs, and unresolved conflicts. These three factors are interrelated. A marriage that lacks mutuality and has numerous unresolved conflicts can in turn discourage feelings of emotional closeness between partners.

Certain changes made by the respondents were occurring that seemed to move them from one phase to the next in the disaffection process. The disaffected spouses were more often attributing marital problems only to the partner, they were putting their own happiness as a higher priority in the relationship, and they were pursuing alternatives to the marriage—either new relationships or other activities.

A Comparison of Disaffected
and Nondisaffected Spouses

The previous chapters included the accounts of spouses who were experiencing disaffection in their marriages. In this chapter we will examine how disaffected spouses differ from nondisaffected spouses on such variables as psychological well-being, commitment, sources of marital problems, and gender. We will be moving beyond qualitative information from a small sample of spouses into the realm of quantitative data collected from a larger survey sample.

The random sample consisted of 354 married individuals who responded to a mailed questionnaire. (See Appendix A for the questionnaire.) The questionnaire was sent to equal numbers of men and women but not to both spouses in the same marriage. Due to the nature of the questions, I thought it was ethically sound to avoid a situation in which spouses could compare their answers, a situation that could increase marital discord. Of course, this meant that I was unable to look at the similarities and discrepancies between the responses of a married couple. But that was not the primary focus of this study.

The sample for the mailed questionnaire was obtained by utilizing the city directories of two Midwestern cities.[1] By selecting the sample from city directories, a broad range of individuals with marriages of various durations and levels of stability was obtained. Fifty-nine percent of the respondents were females, and 41% were males. Their ages ranged from 21 to 84 years old, with a mean age of 46.2 years. The length of marriage ranged from 1 to 58 years, with a mean length of 20.8 years. About 17% of the respondents had been married previously, and approximately 80% had children from their current marriage. The average yearly joint income was $50,000 to $59,999; the average education level was "college graduate."[2]

Marital Disaffection and Psychological Well-Being

Does staying in an unhappy marriage affect the well-being of the individual spouses? What impact does marital disaffection have on a person's emotional well-being? Marriage has the potential to provide much personal happiness in the form of acceptance, love, and support. Therefore, it is expected that individuals experiencing marital disaffection will be deprived of such benefits and, as a consequence, will experience lower personal well-being. The pejorative effects of a marital breakup on one's sense of well-being are quite evident. But could remaining in an emotionally decayed marriage without actually terminating it be equally distressful?

An abundance of data suggests that in general the psychological well-being of married individuals is much better than the unmarried. Compared to unmarried individuals, married individuals experience lower rates of treatment for mental illness (Gove, 1972), higher psychological well-being and overall life satisfaction (Campbell, Converse, & Rodgers, 1976; Gove, Hughes, & Style, 1983; Gove & Shin, 1989; Ryan & Hughes, 1989; Willits & Crider, 1988), and better physical health (Hafner & Miller, 1991). This relationship between marital status and psychological well-being is even stronger for men than for women (Bernard, 1982; Gove, Style, & Hughes, 1990; Gurin, Veroff, & Feld, 1960; Vanfossen, 1986).

But being married in itself does not guarantee emotional well-being. As the accounts in previous chapters convey, not all marriages enhance the spouse's self-concept and self-esteem. Indeed, there is much evidence that marital happiness is more strongly related to psychological well-being than marital status per se (Gove et al., 1983). For example, in their research on married women, O'Connor and Brown (1984) found that the quality of support and the ability to confide in one's husband are important factors in the woman's mental health. Thus, the *quality* of the close relationship, not marital status, makes a difference in mental health. Similarly, Vanfossen (1986), in her study of marriage and depression, found that the social support from one's partner has a significant effect on a spouse's well-being. Affirmation, that is, the degree to which spouses appreciate each other and bring out the the best qualities in each, is the most important type of support for emotional well-being—particularly for wives. Another study revealed that a confiding, intimate relationship with a spouse increases one's ability to cope (Kessler & Essex, 1982). Having an intimate relationship strongly enhances two internal resources, self-esteem and one's sense of mastery, both of which are critical to effective coping.

As expected, when comparing the psychological well-being of disaffected spouses with nondisaffected spouses in the random sample survey, there is an inverse correlation between disaffection and psychological well-being ($r = -.48, p < .001$).[3] When looking at the influence of disaffection along with other variables, such as education, the presence of children, commitment, age, previous marriage, income, and length of marriage, marital disaffection is the strongest negative indicator of psychological well-being ($\beta = -.486, p < .001$). Indeed, this finding supports the importance of a loving marriage to one's sense of well-being.

Let us take a closer look at how a disaffected marriage is related to a person's psychological well-being. The hallmark of a disaffected marriage is the lack of the feeling of love. More specifically, the items defining disaffection include the absence of caring, the lack of an attachment, and little desire for intimacy with one's spouse. Since disaffection is inversely related to psychological well-being, we can conclude that these types of affective or expressive attributes (caring, attachment, intimacy) in marriage are the factors strongly related to psychological well-being. Other researchers (cf. Gove et al., 1990; Heim & Snyder, 1991) have also found a similar relationship between the intimate and expressive aspects of the marital relationship and an individual's well-being. Heim & Snyder (1991) found that marital disaffection, defined as emotional distance and alienation in marriage, is the single best predictor of depression for both husbands and wives. The caring and intimacy felt in a marriage gives spouses a sense of unconditional acceptance and validation that in return enhances their self-concept and emotional well-being. When these factors are missing, as in a disaffected marriage, the consequence is a lower sense of well-being.

The emotional or affective bond in marriage is especially critical in today's society. Whereas in earlier generations, emotional and social support were distributed among others in the community or the extended family, in contemporary society people rely heavily on their partners to provide them with emotional sustenance (Gove et al., 1990, Kersten & Kersten, 1988). More pressure is being placed on the marital relationship to provide for the emotional needs of the individual. Therefore, when these needs are not being met in the marital relationship, it is possible that they will not be met at all.

The relationship between marital disaffection and poor well-being can also be explained from a role theory perspective. If an individual is reasonably successful in his or her major role relationships, such as the marital role, those roles generally will enhance his or her well-being. However, when an individual feels that he or she has failed in the marital role, the individual may experience a poor concept of self, low self-esteem, a sense of incompetence, and a particularly poor state of well-being (Thoits, 1985). It is plausible that the disaffected spouses in my study interpreted the lack of love in their marriages as a personal failure in their role as a spouse.

Commitment and Marital Disaffection

Certainly the role of commitment is critical to the maintenance of a marriage. In Chapter 1 we reviewed some of the literature on commitment and found that commitment is strongly related to the rewards in the relationship, alternative relationships, and costs incurred by leaving the marriage. But when the love and the emotional bond between spouses become tenuous, maintaining one's commitment to the marriage can be a challenge.

Commitment in marriage is not unidimensional: There are different types of commitment. The typology used in this study distinguished between two types of commitment—institutional and voluntary commitment (Blumstein & Schwartz, 1983). A couple with an institutional commitment views marriage as an institution based on a lifetime commitment. Even though the marriage may become unfulfilling, they should persevere and not break the commitment to this institution. In contrast, a couple with a voluntary commitment believes that while the institution may be important, what is more important is how the partners feel about each other and their personal happiness. For these latter couples, marriage must prove itself almost on a daily basis. When a marriage no longer fulfills the spouses' emotional needs, they believe its continuation should be seriously reevaluated. Three items developed by Blumstein and Schwartz (1983) (see Appendix A, Part IV) were used to measure expectations for marital permanence. The responses are summed to form a total score. A high score on these items indicated a belief that marriage should involve a voluntary commitment, and a low score indicated a belief that marriage should involve an institutional commitment.

I wanted to explore further the role of the type of marital commitment in disaffection. Would spouses experiencing disaffection rate lower on commitment? And if so, what type of commitment would they be low on? Some studies suggest that "personal commitment," which is similar to voluntary commitment, is positively related to marital satisfaction (Rollins & Cannon, 1974) and the expression of love (Swensen & Moore, 1979; Swensen et al., 1981). Based on the previous research findings, one could expect that spouses who are high on voluntary commitment would be low on marital disaffection. Perhaps voluntary spouses would believe in a commitment to a relationship that is based solely on feelings toward each other and each other's personal happiness. Not taking the partner or marriage for granted, these spouses would work toward maintaining the love and happiness in marriage (or else leave it). On the other hand, institutional spouses may not work as hard at maintaining love since their marriage is based on a lifetime commitment regardless of its personal fulfillment.

The results of my analysis yielded the opposite finding. A

stepwise multiple regression was performed with marital disaffection as the dependent variable and commitment, as well as other factors, as independent variables. Voluntary commitment was a strong positive indicator of marital disaffection ($\beta = .187, p < .001$), and institutional commitment was not positively correlated with marital disaffection. Therefore, spouses who believe in marriage as a lifelong commitment (an "indissolvable lifetime contract") are less likely to experience marital disaffection.

There are several explanations for this finding. First, there may be factors intrinsic to the type of commitment that could encourage or discourage marital disaffection. Personality traits of persons who make voluntary commitments to marriage may involve a cautiousness about relationships and distrust about people. Their commitment is somewhat tentative. Institutional couples tend to be more trusting and more committed to monogamy than voluntary couples (Blumstein & Schwartz, 1983). For example, the institutional couples are more likely to pool their incomes. "Only couples who are committed to the institution of marriage, not simply to each other, feel safe enough to be able to trust their resources to one another" (Blumstein & Schwartz, 1983, p. 105). Therefore, traits inherent in the personalities of people who make an institutional commitment—such as trust and faithfulness—can help preserve and maintain the affectional bond in the marriage. Perhaps institutional couples treat the marital relationship more seriously and make every effort to take care of it—after all they view their marriage as a commitment for life!

Second, the finding could be explained by cognitive dissonance theory. The theory of cognitive dissonance postulates that people are motivated to maintain a consistency among pairs of relevant cognitions, that is, some belief about themselves, their behavior, or the environment (Campbell, 1987). Since dissonance can be "psychologically uncomfortable," individuals are compelled to reduce the dissonance by altering one of the dissonant cognitions or in some way producing cognitive activity designed to reduce the dissonance. To maintain some consonance between a person's marital commitment and perception of his or her marriage, the individual who believes in marriage as a lifetime commitment also believes that he or she loves his or her spouse since they are staying together for life. In other words, the belief that one loves one's spouse is consistent with the belief that one is staying with that person for life. A person who believes in marriage as a lifelong commitment but does not love his or her partner will need to produce some explanation for his or her lifelong commitment to their partner in order to deal with dissonance. One way to deal with the dissonance is to convince oneself and others that one really does love one's spouse.

Third, the finding may be related to different marital expectations for voluntary couples and institutional couples. Voluntarily committed spouses may have higher expectations than institutionally committed spouses. Voluntary commitment is conditional—the relationship only continues if it meets the spouses' expectations of personal happiness. With high expectations for personal happiness in their marriage, voluntarily committed individuals may become more easily disillusioned with the partner when happiness is not forthcoming. As Bardwick (1979) suggests, "happiness is a fantasy image which denies the constraints imposed by living . . . when expectations are enormously discrepant from reality, goals are unachievable" (p. 120). Expecting their marriages and partners to bring them personal happiness may result in disaffection with the marriage and partner when this goal is not realized. In contrast, the institutionally committed spouses may not be seeking personal fulfillment and happiness in their marital relationship. They may be more satisfied with a relationship that offers them a sense of security and stability.

Finally, voluntary spouses may be more closely monitoring the relationship with increased sensitivity to problems, conflicts, and flaws in the partner. They cannot afford to gloss over problems but need to deal with them in order to ensure their personal happiness. Spouses with the voluntary commitment evaluate the marital relationship with regard to whether it fulfills needs or desires for personal happiness and whether it should be maintained. As we heard in the disaffected spouses' descriptions of the middle phase of disaffection, the overattentiveness to negative traits of the partner can overshadow positive aspects of the relationship and contribute to the growth of disaffection.

Attributions in Marital Relationships

Where spouses place the blame for their marital problems significantly affects their feelings about their marriage. Attribution theory is primarily concerned with people's cognitive explanations of human behavior. Attributions provide an explanation for the behavior of others, upon which we make decisions about how to react toward and make predictions about the future behavior of others (Eiser, 1983). For example, a person's rude and inconsiderate behavior may be attributed to an external event (she's under stress at work) or internal factor (she is an uncaring person). How we explain this behavior will influence our response to the person. With an external explanation we may attempt to be emotionally supportive and empathic to the person under stress. With an internal explanation, we may choose to avoid the person and withdraw. Therefore, the types of attributions about interpersonal behavior that people make will influence their actions and decisions about their relationships, even such major decisions as whether or not to stay in a relationship.

During times of instability in a relationship, attributional activity will be more frequent and will most likely affect the development of the relationship. For example, thinking about the relationship is very frequent during the early stages when important decisions are being made about the relationship (Fletcher, Fincham, Cramer, & Heron, 1987). Another time for increased cognitive activity is when the relationship is perceived as unstable, and separation is under consideration. In such circumstances, there is a high level of motivation to explain the behavior of the partner. Indeed, forming an explanation for the breakup of a relationship can be part of the recovery process when relationships dissolve. Such explanations can serve as a way to maintain one's self-esteem. This is common during the process of disaffection when the relationship is perceived by the disaffected spouse as breaking down and at risk of dissolving.

In recent years, there has been a tremendous increase in the application of attribution theory to the study of close relationships. The role of attributions has been studied in the areas of marital distress (Fincham, 1985; Fincham & Beach, 1988; Fincham & O'Leary, 1983; Holtzworth-Munroe & Jacobson, 1985; Jacobson, McDonald, Follette, & Berley, 1985), marital dissolution (Fletcher, 1983; Harvey, Wells, & Alveraz, 1978), marital conflict (Howe, 1987), marital violence (Andrews & Brewin, 1990), and postdivorce adaptation (Newman, 1981).

In this survey study, I examined the relationship between the level of marital disaffection and the types of attributions used to explain marital problems. Forty-six items of possible sources for marital problems were listed in the survey questionnaire. Respondents were asked to indicate to what extent each item had accounted for problems in their marriage. (See Appendix A, Part II.) These items were categorized by types of attributions: (1) extradyadic, (2) partner, (3) self, and (4) interactive. Extradyadic attributions were those made to events and people outside the dyad and included such items as "moving to a new residence," "financial problems," and "birth of first child."

Partner and self attributions were those explanations that point primarily to characteristics of *either* the partner or the self. The partner attributions included items such as "my spouse's lack of self-disclosure," "my spouse's selfishness," and "my spouse's aggressiveness." Self attributions were the same as the partner attribution items except that they referred to the respondent. An example of a self attribution is, "my own lack of self-disclosure." Interactive attributions were those that point to features of the interaction of the couple. They consisted of such items as "the way my spouse and I solve disagreements," "an unequal distribution of power," and "inadequate communication."

It was hypothesized that marital disaffection would correlate more strongly with partner attributions than to extradyadic, self, or interactive attributions. When analyzing the relationship of marital disaffection to all the types of attributions, the partner and inter-active attributions were the strongest factors in marital disaffection (β's $= .562$ and $.283$, respectively, $p < .001$). Extradyadic attribu-tions were inversely correlated with disaffection ($\beta = -.188$, $p < .001$), meaning that people who were less likely to be disaffected tended to attribute marital problems to extradyadic factors.

The strong association between marital disaffection and part-ner attributions is consistent with previous studies of distressed couples, studies in which the partner was more likely to be blamed for marital problems or marital separation than external circum-stances or the self (Fincham, 1985; Fletcher, 1983; Jacobson et al., 1985). Furthermore, distressed spouses were more willing to dis-credit positive spouse behavior by attributing it to factors outside the partner's personality (Fincham & O'Leary, 1983; Jacobson et al., 1985). In contrast, nondistressed couples were more likely to attrib-ute their partners' positive behavior to internal factors and their negative behavior almost equally to internal and external factors (Jacobson et al., 1985). The external factors studied by Jacobson and his colleagues were similar to the extradyadic factors that I studied, factors that I also found to be used by the nondisaffected spouses in explaining marital problems.

Apparently, among distressed or disaffected spouses, blaming the partner plays a self-serving purpose by alleviating some personal guilt or responsibility for marital problems. Obviously, among dis-affected spouses, marital problems cannot always be the other per-son's fault. Rather it is the *perception* of one spouse that the other is to blame. A striking example of this type of perception is illustrated in Kinsey's research on sexual behavior. Respondents in marriages involving extramarital sex were asked if the extramarital sex caused their divorce. A majority of the respondents stated that their own extramarital sex had *no* effect at all on their divorce. All of the respondents, however, stated that their partner's extramarital sex had an effect on causing the divorce (Kinsey, Pomeroy, Martin, & Gebhard, 1953). Similarly, a more recent study (Buunk, 1987) found that both men and women tend to blame their partner's extradyadic sexual involvements for their relationship breakups more than their own extradyadic relationships. This tendency was more common among the men in the study, who attributed their breakups three times as often to their partner's extradyadic relationships as to their own. Frequent attributions of blame may help spouses deal with their responsibility for marital problems in a face-saving way. But if the blaming is also being expressed to the partner, it can lead to negative reciprocity and conflict escalation.

Regarding the relationship of interactive attributions to marital disaffection, other researchers have found that distressed couples were more likely than nondistressed couples to make interactive attributions, also referred to as relationship attributions (Camper, Jacobson, Holtzworth-Munroe, & Schmaling, 1988; Fincham, 1985). However, there is not always a clear distinction between attributions that focus on the partner and those that are truly dyadic. Fincham (1985) defines a relationship attribution as one in which each partner makes an equal contribution (e.g., "because we trust one another"). In a relationship attribution, *both* spouses are "causal agents" (Howe, 1987). It is not the same as Newman's (1981) interpersonal attribution, which is the perception of the partner in regard to the self (e.g., "She or he does not trust *me*"). Regarding this type of interpersonal attribution, Fincham (1985) states, "To the extent that such ratings reflect partner-oriented attributions, one might expect them to correlate positively with partner blame, whereas truly relationship attributions should not be related to partner blame" (p. 188).

The items used to measure interactive attributions in the present study attempted to reflect attributions in which each partner is sharing responsibility for marital problems. However, similar to Fincham's study, my results revealed a significantly high correlation between the interactive attributions and partner attributions. Perhaps these two types of attributions are highly correlated because they both imply that the spouse does not have unilateral control over the marital problems—responsibility is shared with the partner.

Although partner and interactive attributions may be related, in terms of repairing a relationship, it is important to distinguish them. If a spouse relies almost exclusively on partner attributions for explaining marital problems, they may not be able to see their own contribution to marital problems and be willing to work on making changes themselves. In any case, more research is needed on this question of a distinction between partner and interactive attributions.

Does the relationship between the type of attribution and disaffection apply equally to men and women? Analyses were conducted to look at the influence of these attributions on marital disaffection for males and females separately. The partner attributions again were strong indicators of marital disaffection for both men and women. However, there was a significant difference between men and women on the interactive attributions. While interactive attributions were strong indicators of marital disaffection for women, they did not emerge as a significant factor for men. Since females tend to engage in more relational thinking than men (Acitelli, 1992), it is not surprising that disaffected females were more likely than disaffected males to utilize interactive attributions in explaining marital problems. This finding was consistent with Fincham's (1985) study, which found a tendency for females who were experiencing marital distress to report more relationship attributions.

In my study, overall, men and women reported on average the same number of sources of marital problems. However, I found significant differences between the men and women on the individual items listed in the questionnaire. Significant gender differences appeared on five attribution items. Females were significantly more likely than males to report that their marital problems were the result of their spouse's selfishness, passivity, withdrawal, and substance abuse; their own depressed moods; and an unequal distribution of power. While not significant differences, there was a trend for women to be more likely to report their spouse's emotional immaturity and their lack of motivation to improve the marriage as contributing to the marital problems. Males, more than females, tended to attribute marital problems to their other interests outside the marriage. The tendency for husbands to be more frequently blamed for marital problems was consistent with the national survey conducted by Veroff et al., (1981). These researchers found that "women are much more likely than men to say that their marriage problem stems from some characteristic or problem behavior of their husbands whereas men more often attribute the problem to themselves" (p. 175). In particular, men attributed their own inadequacy as spouses to their lack of sensitivity and responsiveness, while women attributed men's inadequacy to their dominance or bossiness (Veroff et al., 1981).

Does a spouse's attributions for marital problems cause his or her love to decline? Or does the amount of love influence the type of attributions used by a spouse? The direction of causality between attributions and marital disaffection may be difficult to determine from the present survey results. However, findings from recent experiments, treatment outcome studies, and longitudinal studies suggest that attributions are more likely to influence perceived relationship satisfaction than relationship satisfaction affecting the types of attributions (Bradbury & Fincham, 1990).

Gender and Marital Disaffection

The woman cries before the wedding and the man after.
—Polish Proverb

Whoso is tired of happy days let him take a wife.
—Dutch Proverb

Bigamy is having one wife too many. Monogamy is the same.
—British Joke (19th Century)

While popular culture communicates that marriage is an unhappy state for men, the empirical literature suggests otherwise. Numerous studies have found that married women are more likely than married men to be depressed, to be unhappy with their marriages, and to have a negative self-concept (Bernard, 1982; Gove, 1972; Gurin et al., 1960; Pearlin, 1975). Bernard (1982) documents extensively the poor mental and emotional health of married women compared to the health not only of married men but also of unmarried women. She attributes the difference to the enormous adjustments that women make when they marry—adjustments that produce psychological and emotional costs and, over time, increased unhappiness. The survey data in the present study revealed that most spouses still love their partner and that only a minority (19%) feel even some degree of marital disaffection. However, of the group, women are more likely to rate higher on marital disaffection than men ($r = .11, p < .02$).

The differential rate of disaffection among men and women can in part be explained by women's dissatisfaction with the level of intimacy in their marital relationships. Clearly, emotional intimacy is an area of marital interaction in which the sexes diverge.

Men are more likely than women to name their spouses as a confidant and best friend (Lee, 1988; Rubin, 1983). Women perceive less emotional and social support in marriage than men (Depner & Ingersoll-Dayton, 1985; Vanfossen, 1986). Among black women, only about one third report that they would go to their husbands first for support if they had a serious problem such as depression or anxiety (Brown & Gary, 1985). An overwhelming majority of respondents in Hite's (1987) study of 4,500 women state that they are lonely in their heterosexual relationships, experiencing painful and infuriating attitudes on the part of their spouses and giving more emotional support than they are receiving from their men. It is not surprising that many of these women would experience disaffection.

The perceived inequities in marriage for women are another reason for the greater likelihood of disaffection among women. In a longitudinal study of equity and satisfaction in intimate relationships (Van Yperen & Buunk, 1990), spouses were asked to assess what they put into and get out of their relationship compared to what their partners put into and get out of it, and then to evaluate how their relationship "stacks up." More women then men felt underbenefitted, particularly in terms of commitment to the relationship, sociability, and attentiveness. In these areas, women reported that they contribute significantly more than men. At the first interview, twice as many women as men felt deprived in their relationship; in interviews one year later, twice as many men felt overbenefitted. Again, in trying to determine the direction of causality of the relationship between equity and satisfaction, the authors concluded that among women the perception of equity appears to be a better predictor of relationship satisfaction than satisfaction is a predictor of equity (Van Yperen & Buunk, 1990).

In another study (Vanfossen, 1986) which compared four groups of spouses (employed husbands, unemployed husbands, employed wives, and unemployed wives), reciprocity and equity were particularly important to the employed wives. The sense of mastery of these women declined and depression increased when they experienced inequitable relationships with their husbands. In particular, the authors investigated the influence of different types of social support on the wives' well-being. The type of support that proved to enhance wives' self-esteem and buffer them from depression was affirmation, that is, being shown appreciation, having their best qualities brought out, being helped to become the person they would like to be. Interestingly, for women this type of support was more important than what the authors called intimacy, that is, having a confidant or sympathetic listener.

The unequal division of family work continues to be a source of dissatisfaction for women. Wives typically do much more household work and child care than husbands (Warner, 1986), and the notion that women should be responsible for family work and men should "help out" still prevails (Szinovacz, 1984). In general, very few changes in the division of domestic work between husbands and wives have been made over the past decades, leading some researchers to claim that the division of household work is about the same now as it was in the 19th century (Cowan, 1987). For example, between 1965 and 1975 husbands' time in household work and child care did not change even though there was a decline in their time in paid work. It is believed that husbands spent their extra time in leisure (Coverman & Sheley, 1986).

As can be expected, husbands who are in marriages with these inequities in housework and child care are more satisfied with their marriages and less critical of their wives, while the women are less satisfied (Barnett & Baruch, 1987; Benin & Agostinelli, 1988; Yogev & Brett, 1985). Conversely, wives with husbands who do their share of family work are more satisfied with marriage than other wives (Staines & Libby, 1986) and evaluate their husbands less critically (Barnett & Baruch, 1987). In Vanfossen's (1986) study of women and depression, many of the women were experiencing role overload because of their dual roles as employee and housekeeper. Wives who felt overwhelmed by their duties, who perceived their husbands as demanding and unwilling to help in matters in the home, and who had conflict with their husbands over these conditions were particularly likely to be depressed (Vanfossen, 1986).

These continuing inequities in family work contribute to the disaffection among women. The unfairness reflects an uncaring and demeaning attitude of men toward women. The message communicated to women is that they should serve the needs or demands of husbands over their own. Perhaps this is what Bernard (1982) meant by "dwindling" into a wife. Hence, it is understandable how resentment may grow and loving feelings toward the husband diminish in such inequitable relationships.

Although the likelihood of experiencing disaffection in marriage is different for men and women, when disaffection is experienced, it impacts men's and women's psychological well-being equally. No significant differences in disaffection and well-being for men and women were found in my study. While there has been a recent emphasis on the importance of close relationships and "connections" in women's development of self (Gilligan, 1982; Jack, 1991; Jordan et al., 1991), the importance of close relationships to the well-being of men should not be minimized. Indeed, much of the research on well-being and marital status has found that unmarried men are worse off than married men in terms of mental and physical health (Gove et al., 1990). While these data do not provide information on the quality of these marriages—only their marital status is reported—they, nonetheless, emphasize the importance of marital relationships to men. Both men and women seek similar rewards in marriage—love, affection, emotional support, companionship, and intimacy. Because a person's sense of self and well-being are promoted or enhanced from the satisfaction of these needs, when they are not met, as in a disaffected relationship, psychological well-being will be negatively affected. Men and women may differ in the way they express intimacy, but the desires and needs for a close, self-enhancing relationship exist for both sexes.

Summary

In a comparison of disaffected and nondisaffected spouses, my data revealed that disaffected spouses were more likely to rate lower on psychological well-being, believe in voluntary commitment to marriage, use partner and interactive attributions for marital problems, and be female. When a spouse is experiencing marital disaffection, it is likely that the aspects of a relationship that are enhancing to a person's well-being—caring, attachment, and intimacy—are missing. Of course, it is also possible that an individual's well-being affects his or her feelings toward the partner. If a person feels depressed and unhappy personally, he or she may perceive the marriage and the partner negatively. Although the direction of causality between disaffection and psychological well-being cannot be clearly determined, a likely explanation is that being in a loveless marriage affects a person's happiness and well-being rather than vice versa.

The relationship between individuals who strongly believe in an institutional commitment (i.e., marriage as an "indissolvable lifetime contract") and lower rates of marital disaffection can be explained by several theories. First, there may be some factors intrinsic to the institutional commitment that may discourage marital disaffection from occurring. Second, cognitive dissonance theory suggests that individuals have a need to create consonance between the beliefs of a lifetime commitment and stating their love for their spouse. Third, voluntary couples and institutional couples may have different marital expectations. Spouses with a voluntary commitment may have higher expectations and be particularly vigilant of marital problems and flaws of the partner.

Disaffected spouses were more likely than nondisaffected spouses to place blame for marital problems on the partner and the interaction of the spouses. The extensive use of partner attributions by disaffected spouses plays a self-serving purpose in alleviating some personal guilt or responsibility for marital problems. Again, the direction of causality is difficult to determine, but based on some previous longitudinal research, it appears that frequent blaming of the partner leads to disaffection rather than disaffection producing partner attributions for problems. Similarly, in the interviews with the disaffected spouses, partner attributions were frequently used in the beginning of the process of disaffection and seemed to add fuel to the growing disaffection.

Females tended to experience marital disaffection more frequently than males. This finding is consistent with previous research on marital satisfaction that has found that men are generally happier in their marriages than women. Reasons for women's unhappiness include their dissatisfaction with the amount of emotional intimacy in their marriage and the overall inequities in the marital relationship. Further analyses of gender differences uncovered that the psychological well-being of males and females was similarly affected by marital disaffection. Apparently, disaffection has the same impact on well-being regardless of whether you are male or female. One gender difference that emerged was that females were more likely to use interactive attributions in explaining their marital problems. Given their greater propensity for relational thinking, it is not surprising that women would more frequently than men attribute problems to the interaction of the couple.

In general, the findings of the random sample survey were very similar to the findings from the in-depth interviews conducted with disaffected spouses. Like the survey findings, the interviews revealed the negative effects of disaffection on well-being and the frequent use of partner attributions during the process of disaffection. Because there were fewer males than females interviewed, it is difficult to get a clear picture of gender differences from the interviews. Perhaps the overwhelming response of disaffected women to my advertisements for the study provides further support for the finding that disaffection is more commonly experienced by women than men.

Notes

1. A systematic sampling procedure was used in the survey. The number of married couples in these directories was estimated and then divided by 800—the approximate total number of questionnaires that I wanted to send out. The resulting number was 28. The starting point was designated by choosing a random number between 1 and 28. Then every 28th married couple after that number was chosen. Since only one spouse from each couple was selected for the survey, I alternated between choosing a husband or wife. A recurring pattern of every 28th married couple in the directory does not appear to bias the sample in any way. The final total of married individuals selected from the directories was 752.

Forty-five of the questionnaires could not be delivered because the potential respondents had moved without leaving forwarding addresses. An additional 35 questionnaires were sent to individuals who were no longer married due to divorce or death. It is possible there may have been more of these individuals, but these 35 telephoned or wrote back indicating that they were no longer married.

Postcards accompanied the questionnaire sent to each potential respondent. The card was to be signed and sent to me, separate from the questionnaire, when the respondent completed and sent in his or her questionnaire. If after 3 weeks from when the questionnaires were mailed this postcard was not received, a reminder postcard was mailed. A letter with a replacement questionnaire was sent to non-respondents 4 weeks after the follow-up postcard.

2. The average joint income of the survey respondents ($50,000–$59,999) was higher than the estimated average household income for the two cities (*Editor and Publisher Market Guide*, 1988). It may be that higher-income individuals are more likely to respond to a mailed questionnaire dealing with marriage.

Likewise, the survey respondents tended to be more highly educated than average; 56% of the sample were college graduates compared to 40% of the total population (25 years and over) of the two cities (U.S. Bureau of the Census, 1980). Since the 1980 Census Bureau statistic is outdated, the current percentage of college graduates could be somewhat higher, but it is likely that college graduates may be more prone to respond to a mailed questionnaire on marriage and that the sample may be somewhat biased in this direction.

3. A list of nine feelings taken from R. Miller (1982) (see Appendix A, Part III) was used to measure psychological well-being. The respondent indicated to what degree each feeling applied to him or her. Possible answers ranged from 1 = "Not at all" to 10 = "A lot."

$S \cdot E \cdot V \cdot E \cdot N$

Restoring Love
in a Disaffected Marriage

*When we started counseling, the first time we came I had had
it in my mind that the marriage was going to end. I mean this
was a last-ditch effort. I had already made it up in my mind
that this marriage was not going to work and this was my last
attempt.*

(26-year-old female, married 6 years)

As we have seen in previous chapters, marital disaffection exacts a
high cost on psychological well-being and is a common source of
emotional distress. Furthermore, if marital disaffection results in
divorce, social, emotional, and economic consequences are experienced by *both* spouses and children. Despite the high psychological and social costs, most couples experiencing marital distress do
not seek formal help in dealing with it. When help is sought, very
few spouses consult mental health professionals, instead they bring
their problems to the clergy and family physicians (Veroff, Kulka,
& Douvan, 1981). Even divorcing spouses during the year prior to
filing for divorce are almost as likely to seek help from a physician
or member of the clergy as from a mental health professional
(psychiatrist, psychologist, marriage counselor, or social worker)
(Kitson, 1992).

The purpose of this chapter is to present clinical interventions
that assist in treating marriages in which at least one partner is
experiencing marital disaffection. Although the chapter will focus
on marital therapy, we must remember that there are couples who

regain their love without professional intervention. A recent study (Mackey & O'Brien, 1992) revealed that many couples of long-term marriages are able to solve their problems on their own or through nonprofessional support. The researchers of this study concluded that many "indigenous services"—such as religious or community groups—can serve as alternatives to professional psychotherapy in helping distressed couples.

The interventions proposed in this chapter are organized around the three phases of disaffection that have been described in earlier chapters. Understanding the salient issues of each phase of disaffection can assist the practitioner in setting goals and implementing interventions to stop further deterioration and restore the emotional bond. Certain interventions may be particularly helpful at one stage of the disaffection process but ineffective at another stage. For example, interventions that are effective in helping couples deal with early disillusionment with the marriage may not be as helpful at the end of the disaffection process when one partner is seriously contemplating divorce. Therefore, care needs to be taken to determine the phase of disaffection so that the effective interventions can be implemented. While the interventions in this chapter are organized around the phases of disaffection, this is not meant to be a step-by-step cookbook approach to marital therapy. Rather the goal is to assist the clinician in assessing what phase of disaffection the spouses are experiencing and what interventions would be appropriate given the salient issues and relevant goals for the particular phase.

Early Interventions: Preventing Marital Disaffection

The time when couples need help the most is often during the first year of their marriage. Ironically, this is when the least help has traditionally been available. Sixty percent of the disaffected spouses in my study reported marital dissatisfaction and doubts about their marriages during the first year of their marriage. A study of divorced couples across the life cycle found that one third of the couples admitted to having been in serious trouble by the time of their first wedding anniversary (Thornes & Collard, 1979). The most common period for divorce to occur is 2 to 5 years after the marriage. "Given the time required to make the decision to divorce, separate, file, and wait for a final decree, this peak period reflects evidence of serious marital problems very early in the relationship for most couples who eventually divorce" (Spanier & Thompson, 1984, p. 13).

While marital problems may emerge early in a marriage, there has not yet been an extensive history of hurtful and bitter feelings, negative interactions, and dispairing thoughts about the marriage. Therefore, preventive interventions are most effective at the beginning phase of disaffection. David and Vera Mace, founders of the Association of Couples for Marital Enrichment (ACME), concluded that preventive services are critical early in the marriage:

> It just wasn't enough to wait until a couple became seriously alienated, and then try to reverse the degeneration that had been developing over a period of years. Of course we had no other alternative than this for couples who were already in real trouble; but surely, we said, it should be possible to *prevent* the degenerative process by offering help at an earlier stage. In plain English, we must match our *remedial* services with corresponding *preventive* services, thus cutting back on the failure rate. Providing only therapy is like providing only hospitals, and giving people no guidance about how to stay well. (Mace & Mace, 1986, p. 20)

To implement preventive services, the Maces suggested that professional practitioners set up monthly sessions with newlyweds (either as couples or groups of couples) during the first year of marriage. One such program has been put into operation in Kansas City under the name of Growth in Marriage for Newlyweds. This is a 6-week marriage enrichment experience designed especially for couples in their first year of marriage.

Since the Maces' establishment of the Association of Couples for Marriage enrichment, many other psychoeducational groups for couples have been developed. Examples of these programs include

Relationship Enhancement (Guerney, 1977), Couple's Communication Program (Miller, Nunnally, & Wackman, 1976), Marriage Encounter (Gallagher, 1975), and Communication Problem-Solving Workshops (Witkin, Edelson, Rose, & Hall, 1983). A meta-analytic study on these programs concluded that, on average, enrichment programs lead to significant improvements in relationship skills and that these gains are usually maintained for many months (Giblin, Sprenkle, & Sheehan, 1985). However, Doherty, Lester, and Leigh (1986) voice concern about the appropriateness of intensive marital programs, such as Marriage Encounter, for very distressed couples. The results from their study behoove leaders of enrichment programs to carefully screen the degree of distress of couples before recommending such programs. These results also suggest that psychoeducational couples programs may be quite appropriate during the initial phase of disaffection before anger and hurt have escalated.

Unfortunately, research reveals that few couples avail themselves of any kind of professional intervention early in the marriage. The statistics on marital preparation programs are also quite disappointing. Fewer than half of all couples who marry will participate in marital preparation programs (Olson, 1983). More then 60% of the couples offered the premarital program, PREP (Prevention and Relationship Enhancement Program), either declined the treatment or dropped out before completing it (Markman, Duncan, Storaasli, & Howes, 1987).

Couples' hesitation to seek help early in the marriage may be explained in part by the "intermarital taboo" in our culture (Mace & Mace, 1986). This taboo discourages married couples from talking openly to other couples about what is going on in their relationship. Consequently, they have little opportunity to share their difficulties with others and to learn the skills that are needed in an intimate and enduring marital relationship.

> Couples feel quite free to ask each other for help if the flowers in the garden aren't growing properly, or if the dog is sick, or even if the baby is causing trouble. But if their *interpersonal*

relationship isn't working well, that is a *close secret* and you just don't talk about it. Only when the situation is far advanced and desperate is it appropriate to turn to marriage counseling. (Mace & Mace, 1986, p. 20)

Unfortunately, assistance that could prevent problems from escalating into bigger conflicts and greater disaffection is not sought.

A second reason for the reluctance to seek help stems from another cultural myth: A successful marriage should come naturally and effortlessly. Therefore,

To seek assistance for one's marriage, either before or after significant problems have arisen, is to admit that one is inadequate and unsuccessful and that one has failed at what is believed to be a simple task; seeking help is therefore discouraged, and steps to prevent marital dysfunction are compromised. (Bradbury & Fincham, 1990, p. 380)

It also reflects society's idealistic obsession with romantic love—a love that an individual simply falls into and is maintained forever with little effort.

Likewise, professional counselors are probably equally at fault for the lack of attention to early intervention and prevention. Prevention does not attract many mental health professions. It does not offer "clear and lucrative career options, is not glamorous enough, stifles creativity, and is too limited and structured, especially when compared to psychotherapy" (Bradbury & Fincham, 1990, p. 380). More emphasis is placed on treating couples in psychotherapy after long-standing and serious marital distress than on helping to prevent the problems from occurring in the first place.

Early intervention #1: Teaching interpersonal skills. The specific type of intervention that can be most helpful to couples in the first phase of disaffection is social skills training, such as conflict resolution and communication skills (Gottman, Notarius, Gonso, & Markman, 1976; Guerney, 1977; L'Abate, 1977; Miller, Nunnally, & Wackman, 1976; Valle & Marinelli, 1975). These training programs teach spouses to express thoughts and emotions in a clear, direct, and nonhostile manner, and to listen by reflecting an understanding of the other's expressed messages (Baucom & Epstein, 1990). Couples are taught to resolve conflict using a collaborative approach, in contrast with a competitive approach. The advantage of intervention into the marriage at this time is that the union is still young— most likely hostility, anger, and resentment have not built up—but spouses are beginning to see their partners realistically, and conflicts are emerging that were previously glossed over.

Whereas a social skills training approach is effective in teaching skills, sometimes a deficit of skills is not the problem. Rather there are other factors preventing the demonstration of constructive communication and conflict resolution. Spouses may be performing these skills quite adequately with other people but not with their marital partner. In such cases, the clinician may need to examine underlying motivations and factors in the environment that prevent the spouse from utilizing social skills (for example, some punitive consequence from the partner). The intention to perform the behavior is a powerful and immediate factor preceding the actual behavior. Although other factors may influence the success of the attempt, the stronger the intent, the more successful the outcome. "To the extent that the individual has the opportunity and the resources to perform a behavior, the theory of planned behavior predicts that intent to perform the behavior is the primary variable determining extent of success" (Beach, 1991, p. 314). An individual's intent is closely tied to the belief that the behavior is linked to some positive or negative outcome. If a spouse believes that complying with a particular therapeutic directive will result in negative consequences, it is likely that he or she would not comply (Beach, 1991).

A spouse's intention may be the strongest during the beginning phase of marital disaffection, and then it weakens with the onset of hostile, angry feelings and thoughts of ending the marriage. During the beginning phase of disaffection, the respondents recalled feeling quite hopeful that the relationship would change and the marriage would work out. At this point, a therapist can take advantage of the hopeful feelings to elicit the spouse's cooperation in learning and performing new skills. Later, as hope dwindles, it is more difficult because the spouse does not foresee that complying with the therapist's directives will make any difference in the marriage. (Note the pessimism in the quote at the beginning of this chapter.) Therefore, it is important to consider the following factors influencing compliance to a social skills training approach: (1) the attitude toward the behavior, including the individual's perceived consequences of engaging in the behavior, (2) the social pressure felt by the individual, including his or her degree of motivation to conform to the expectations of these significant others, and (3) the individual's perception that he or she can perform the behavior, including the necessary opportunities, and the required resources to perform the skills (Beach, 1991).

Early intervention #2: Addressing marital expectations. A second area of focus during this initial phase is an examination of marital expectations. The disillusionment that was frequently described during the beginning phase of disaffection was often the result of the partners and the marriage not meeting preconceived expectations. Spouses enter their marriage with a set of expectations of their mate and what they wish to give to the relationship. There is some empirical evidence that never-married individuals have much higher and unrealistic expectations for marriage than married individuals (Sabatelli, 1988). Therefore, spouses need to reevaluate their expectations for marriage after getting married if they are to continue to be satisfied with their relationship.

Sager (1981) conceptualizes these expectations as "marital contracts." In the beginning of the couple's relationship these "marital contracts" are mostly unexpressed. But as conflicts in the relationship emerge, they need to be explored and brought to the awareness of the partners. Part of the illusionary intimacy described in Chapter 2 is the assumption that both partners subscribe to the same unspoken set of terms for the relationship. An example of a conflicting contract is one in which one spouse expects never to be lonely and to always have the partner present as a companion, while the other spouse expects marriage to allow freedom to pursue individual interests and other relationships. Hence, much of the clinical work with couples at this early juncture of marriage involves helping a couple arrive at *one* functioning contract—the terms of which both partners are aware of and can subscribe to.

In a similar vein, Baucom and Epstein (1990) refer to these individual contracts as personal *standards* about how a "good" marriage should be. It is the *combination* of two spouses' standards that often produces problems. An illustration of conflicting standards is a case in which one spouse thinks that in a good marriage spouses avoid having disagreements while the other spouse views a good marriage as one in which the spouses express all of their feelings and opinions to one another (Baucom & Epstein, 1990). These standards can also include role expectations, such as whether one spouse's career will have a higher priority or how the housework will be allocated. Table 7.1 contains a list of common dysfunctional relationship standards.

To help spouses arrive at more realistic relationship standards, Baucom and Epstein (1990) suggest conducting a logical analysis of the standard while gathering evidence about the standard's validity.

TABLE 7.1 Common Dysfunctional Relationship Standards

1. Spouses should be able to sense each other's needs and thoughts as if they could read each other's mind.
2. One should be a perfect sexual partner.
3. In order to demonstrate his/her love, a spouse must (do *X*).
4. Over the course of a relationship, being in love should feel like (some version of "the bells ringing").
5. You do not have to be polite to your partner, as you would be to an acquaintance, friend, or stranger.
6. In a close relationship, spouses should meet all of each other's needs.
7. A person is fully responsible for maintaining his or her spouse's happiness in life.
8. Spouses should be completely supportive of all of each other's ideas and actions.

From Baucom & Epstein (1990, p. 319). Copyright 1990 by D. H. Baucom. Reprinted by permission.

This analysis can include constructing a list of advantages and disadvantages for adhering to these standards. The therapist helps the spouses to rate the importance of each item on the list. The next step is to revise the standard but not totally eliminate it. Baucom and Epstein describe more completely the steps of this intervention in their book *Cognitive-Behavioral Marital Therapy* (1990).

The examination of transgenerational issues may also assist spouses in identifying their expectations for marriage. A spouse may be expecting his or her partner to compensate for what the spouse's parents did not provide in his or her family of origin. Spouses need to sort out what happened in the past in the original family so that the feelings toward and conflicts with their parents do not get displaced and projected onto the marital partner (Paul & Paul, 1986). Spouses, in essence, must achieve an emotional divorce from the original nuclear family before they can make a viable marriage.

Middle Interventions: Reviving the Marriage

By the middle phase of disaffection, the spouse has attempted to communicate his or her dissatisfactions, but significant change has not taken place. This is a critical phase in the process of disaffection. If positive changes are not realized, the disaffected spouse will start to lose hope, and resentment will build. In fact, if there has been extensive hurt already, the disaffected spouse may already be reluctant to work on the marriage in order to avoid further disappointment and hurt should no changes be forthcoming. Such feelings need to be acknowledged in order to convince the spouse to take a risk in improving the relationship. Often disaffected spouses want to wait until their feelings change before attempting to engage in new behaviors. However, it is important that the marital therapist encourages the spouses to adhere to the "as if" principle, that is, act *as if* they have the feelings rather than waiting for the feelings to change first (Stuart, 1980). Stuart (1980) further explains how to address this dilemma with the following advice to marriage counselors:

Distressed family members often complain that their feelings of love for the others have died. They plaintively ask therapists to help restore those treasured feelings before they begin, anew, loving behaviors toward their mates. But feelings of love can grow only through interaction with the other; therefore, the key to relationship change is that the love-lost client must act toward the other as if loving feelings were alive and well, for only then will the other's loving actions be stimulated—actions that can truly support our client's love for his or her mate. Therapeutic behavior change of every sort is therefore seen to depend upon the therapist's skill in encouraging the client's willingness to reach beyond reality and to summon the willingness to act as if the world were a welcoming place, for it must remain the forbidding place it is believed to be until these new behaviors occur. (p. 27)

The hope is that as the partner's behavior changes, the feelings of the disaffected spouse will change. This is not likely to happen immediately, but over time.

Middle intervention #1: Increasing positive exchanges. One goal at this stage is to increase the level of positive behavioral exchanges, while reducing the exchanges of negative, hurtful behaviors. The *maintenance* of any positive changes is crucial. Many of the disaffected spouses in my study stated that the changes made by their partner were very short-lived. The first step in preventing such relapses is teaching spouses how to transform vague descriptions of complaints and dissatisfactions into explicit behaviors. By teaching the couple to pinpoint specific behaviors that they would like changed, the clinician can help to modify and reduce displeasing behaviors. Interventions such as "Caring Days," (Stuart, 1980), "Love Days" (Weiss, Hops, & Patterson, 1973), and behavioral contracts (Jacobson & Margolin, 1979) can be used to increase positive behavior exchanges between the spouses. These interventions are based on social exchange principles that assert that as one spouse demonstrates positive behavior, the partner will reciprocate with a positive action.

To begin the intervention of positive exchange, each spouse is asked to compile a list of requests for small behaviors that convey a feeling of being cared for by the other (Stuart, 1980). "Caring" is a term preferred over "love" because "couples are usually more willing to commit themselves to act as if they care for each other than to act as if they love one another" (p. 199). Stuart further explains:

> Love may or may not be the end point of treatment, but it can never be its start. Thus, delay of confrontation of conflict, adoption of an as-if strategy, and pursuit of caring and tenderness rather than love are a trio of antecedents, the absence of which is very likely to undermine any hope of success through the caring-days technique. (p. 199)

After discussing and agreeing to the items on each other's list, the spouses are asked to carry out these activities. During the week, each spouse is to record on the list of caring acts the date on which he or she received a caring act. Generally, the spouse who is less disaffected will be willing to comply with this effort at change. The disaffected spouse, however, will need some encouragement from the therapist. The therapist can help the disaffected spouse in viewing the caring-days process as a "low-cost method of assessing the feasibility of relationship change" (Stuart, 1980, p. 199).

In addition to change on a behavioral level, keeping track of these positive behavioral exchanges can produce perceptual changes. The caring exchanges may help spouses to notice positive aspects of the partner that had been previously overlooked or discounted during the process of disaffection. The research on attribution theory reveals that distressed couples discredit positive marital events and that perceptual errors occur as spouses scan selectively for negative behaviors of their partner. Keeping a record of caring behaviors, thus, increases spouses' sensitivity and attentiveness to positive events (Baucom & Epstein, 1990).

Middle Intervention #2: Modifying attributions for marital events. During the middle stage, the disaffected spouse tends to blame the partner for most of the marital problems. Earlier in the process, the spouses also blamed themselves and extradyadic factors. But now responsibility for problems shifts primarily to the partner. When spouses blame their partner, they are taking little responsibility for the causes and possible resolutions of their marital problems. Furthermore, if the disaffected spouse is expressing blame to his or her partner, this may lead to negative reciprocity and conflict escalation because it is likely that the partner will respond negatively to the continual blaming. Therefore, the clinician needs to take the focus away from "blaming" the partner exclusively. This requires change on the cognitive level since it is primarily the *perception* of the partner's behavior rather than the *behavior* itself that is producing the dissatisfaction in the relationship (Baucom & Epstein, 1990).

In recent years there has been tremendous growth in the area of marital therapy focused on changing cognitions. Beck (1988) has identified numerous errors in spouses' thinking, such as tunnel vision, selective abstraction, arbitrary inference, overgeneralization, magnification, negative labeling, and biased explanations. Spouses use these cognitive distortions when attempting to explain events that occur in the marriage. For example, tunnel vision means that a spouse is only looking at a particular behavior or event—in the case of disaffection it is usually a negative one—and disregards other facts that may give a more balanced picture of a situation. Cognitive interventions help couples change their perceptual errors and causal attributions in order to feel less angry and distressed about their marriage.

One cognitive strategy developed by Baucom (1987) helps spouses to shift responsibility for problems away from the partner. This technique involves making the attribution process more explicit so that the interpretations being made can be assessed for appropriateness. The intervention involves asking the couple to discuss the causes of and explanations for a problem in their marital relationship and to think of alternative explanations for the situation. The therapist acknowledges that the original attribution is a possible explanation for the event, but he or she emphasizes that it is important to determine whether this is the most accurate or reasonable explanation. The couple is asked how each of the following factors have contributed to the problem: environmental or outside circumstances, husband's behavior, wife's behavior, husband's interpretation of wife's behavior, wife's interpretation of husband's behavior, husband's emotional reaction, and wife's emotional reaction. During this discussion, each spouse focuses on his or her own behavior, thoughts, and emotional reactions. This process broadens both spouses' views of causality in their relationship. As the therapist guides the couple in testing the relative validity of the various alternatives, the couple may come up with another explanation based solely on logical grounds (Baucom & Epstein, 1990).

In order to test the validity or reasonableness of an attribution, the therapist, along with the spouses, gather evidence from a variety of sources. These sources of evidence include: (1) details of the couple's past experiences that contradict current thinking, (2) changes in the couple's behaviors and perceptions of each other over the course of the relationship, (3) written logs and diaries, (4) in vivo marital interactions during conjoint therapy sessions, and (5) planned behavioral experiments. While this examination of evidence can help a couple evaluate the reasonableness of their cognitions, Baucom and Epstein (1990) also suggest guiding them in assessing the usefulness of those attributions. In other words, individuals may hold on to certain attitudes or beliefs (even in the face of contradictory evidence) because they are functional. Therefore, it is necessary to assist the spouses in identifying and weighing the advantages and disadvantages of their attributions and beliefs.

The goal of this intervention is to help spouses recognize multiple factors that contribute to a problem—and the subjective nature of interpretation of the causes of problems—so that the partner is not totally and automatically blamed for the problems. It is hoped that as interpretations for marital events are modified and expanded beyond partner blame, there will be a concomitant increase in positive feelings toward the partner.

Besides changing attributions for problems and negative events in the marriage, the couple and therapist can identify events that highlight the partner's positive behavior, for which the spouse can make positive partner attributions (Baucom, 1987). Attention can be drawn to the positive events in the marriage and the partner's good intentions and positive behaviors. In sum, cognitive marital therapy helps to prevent further growth of disaffection by teaching spouses to reduce their cognitive distortions and negative partner attributions and to develop a more balanced view of the relationship.

End Phase Interventions: The Point of No Return?

End phase intervention #1: Addressing the bitterness. Special interventions during the end phase need to target the long-standing anger and resulting bitterness that are experienced during this phase. Examining bitterness and reducing it is a critical task in repairing a disaffected marriage. If the bitterness goes unaddressed, then the disaffected spouse will be reluctant to take responsibility for himself or herself—an essential step for reconciliation and successful restoration of love (Guerin, Fay, Burden, & Kautto, 1987). Although the partner is possibly making changes in the relationship by this time, the disaffected spouse's bitter feelings may overshadow these changes. Specific therapeutic steps need to be utilized with embittered spouses, especially when the anger and hurts have been long-standing. The following is an overview of steps to help disaffected spouses work through their anger and bitterness. Further elaboration of this "bitterness protocol" is in *The Evaluation and Treatment of Marital Conflict* (Geurin et al., 1987).

1. *Acknowledge the fantasy solution and test its reality.* Because many disaffected spouses give up hope that their spouse will change, they spend a great deal of time absorbed in a fantasy about life without the spouse. They may be fantasizing about their partner dying or their own death. The therapist helps the spouse test the reality of the fantasy by asking questions about what their life would be like without the partner. Instead of confronting the fantasy, the therapist explores the fantasy with the spouse. But the therapist also conveys that it is dysfunctional to spend so much time and energy fantasizing about life without the partner; it is a way to avoid changing oneself.

2. *Identify the "bitter bank" and reframe it as self-destructive.* The "bitter bank" refers to the accumulation of bitterness that builds over time. By the end phase of disaffection, spouses are so focused on their partner as the cause of marital problems that they do not recognize the degree to which bitterness dominates their emotional lives. The intervention at this point is to help the disaffected spouse refocus from the partner to himself or herself. The therapist labels the many complaints about the partner as coming from the spouse's bitter bank. Next, the therapist helps the spouse become aware that bitterness has become a way of life that is more destructive to the spouse himself or herself than to anyone else. The spouse needs to recognize that the time and energy devoted to the bitter bank prevents him or her from developing more productive aspects of life.

3. *Track the bitterness back through the process from disillusionment to disaffection.* The therapist encourages the spouse to tell the story of his or her disaffection. The focus is on the spouse's experience of bitterness, and the message is that the spouse needs to take responsibility for changing the course of his or her feelings.

4. *Examine the bitterness as a generational pattern.* Bitterness in previous generations can cause expectations of marriage that individuals bring into their own marriages. In particular, these individuals may have greater expectations in order to compensate for disappointments of their ancestors. Therefore, the therapist may need to explore with the disaffected spouse whether there was bitterness in his or her family of origin to determine if compensation for others' disappointments is fueling the spouse's current bitterness.

5. *Modify the perception of the victimized spouse.* Often the bitter spouse is viewing himself or herself as a victim of the partner's unrelenting hurtful and controlling behaviors. This step in the bitterness protocol involves helping the embittered spouse identify his or her perception of the enemy–victim behavior pattern, change their own behavior, and evaluate the marital system's response to the change. By analyzing situations in which the bitter spouse acts as a victim, the therapist can encourage alternative responses, such as acting toward the partner in more direct and assertive ways.

Evaluating the partner's response to the new behavior can help the embittered spouse view the impact of his or her new behavior and its effect on developing new patterns of marital interaction.

6. *Work with the emptiness that comes when bitterness is gone.* During the process of disaffection, an inordinate amount of time is spent on thinking about and feeling angry and bitter about the partner and the marriage. Because much time and energy has been spent on bitterness, when it is given up, the individual is likely to feel depleted and drained. At this point, the therapist can help the disaffected spouse describe the emotions he or she is experiencing and replace the old bitter internal dialogues with new, more positive thoughts.

7. *Develop personal goals and work to reach them.* During this step the therapist helps the bitter client to evaluate his or her current level of satisfaction and functioning in the areas of work, other personal relationships, and personal well-being. This may involve encouraging the spouse to define goals for himself or herself and develop a plan for achieving these goals. The therapist may need to focus on any marital or personal factors that inhibit the progress toward these goals.

End phase intervention #2: Working with ambivalence. During the final stage of disaffection many spouses may need to deal with ambivalence about the possible dissolution of the marriage. For the ambivalent spouse, therapy focuses on making a decision about the marriage—either an attempt to repair it or to disengage from it. Kressel (1985) suggests three principal diagnostic issues in this decision-making phase:

1. Is the marital distress primarily a result of problems in the marital relationship or in the personal conflicts of one of the marital partners?
2. Regardless of its locus, is the movement toward divorce a positive or negative development?
3. Regardless of whether the movement toward divorce is positive or negative (from the clinician's perspective), from

a practical point of view, is it too late to do anything about it? (p. 93)

An intervention designed to assist distressed marital couples during the decision-making period is a structured separation (Granvold, 1983). One purpose of such a separation is "to put a sense of choice back into a relationship in which the individuals feel 'stuck' or paralyzed in terms of freely choosing either to be together or to be apart" (Rice & Rice, 1986, p. 285). Overall, the purpose is for the spouses to have time away from each other in order to make a decision about relationship maintenance or termination. A structured separation involves a mutually written agreement specifying the rules and guidelines of the separation. The terms of the contract may include the following items: (1) duration of the separation, (2) frequency of contact between the spouses, (3) sexual contact between the spouses, (4) dating, (5) sexual contact with others, (6) contact with children, (7) financial support, and (8) expectations for ongoing therapy (Granvold, 1983). At the end of the designated length of separation the spouses are asked to agree to participate in renegotiating the separation if there is a desire to continue the separation period.

One limitation of the structured separation is that it requires the cooperation and collaboration of both spouses during a time of emotional upset and stress when cooperation may be most difficult to attain. It is unlikely that both spouses are at the same place in terms of their feelings about the marriage. Given these discrepant feelings, spouses may approach therapy with different agendas, which are likely to lead to frustrated efforts at negotiating a separation (Rice & Rice, 1986). Whereas a structured separation may not effectively prevent a divorce from occurring, there is research suggesting that spouses who carry out a structured separation with counseling experience few difficulties in reaching a divorce settlement (Toomim, 1972).

End phase intervention #3: Helping spouses to disengage. If the disaffected spouse clearly has made a decision to end the marriage, a structured separation will not be a useful intervention. Therefore, the therapist needs to assess carefully the goals and agendas of spouses when they seek counseling.

> One spouse may have decided that he or she wants out of the relationship and may have someone else "waiting in the wings." Primarily out of guilt, such an individual may have come to therapy basically to turn over the spouse to the therapist. Thus, one spouse's hidden agenda may be to get out of therapy as quickly as possible and get on with his or her (other) life. To set up a therapeutic contract to work together (e.g., in a structured separation with counseling) is likely to be unproductive in such circumstances. Hidden agendas of one or both individuals should be brought out into the open as soon as psychologically feasible in therapy, while taking into account what may be the defensive purpose of such behaviors. (Rice & Rice, 1986, pp. 293–294)

The goal of treatment in such cases is not to repair the relationship but to facilitate the disengagement. Persons dissolving their relationship may not have "an effective set of strategies and skills for doing so" (Duck, 1982, p. 29). Therefore, the focus of therapy needs to be on mediation of practical concerns (e.g., financial arrangements, visitation and child-custody arrangements, setting up separate households, facilitating the legal process) and dealing with the postseparation adjustment. Social and psychological issues may involve redefining an identity without the marital partner, dealing with people in the social network, dealing with guilt and a sense of personal failure about ending the marriage, and dealing with anxiety at the prospect of separation. Besides individual counseling, divorce recovery groups can provide a supportive context in which divorcing spouses can deal with many of these issues.

Summary

Repairing a relationship that has gone awry is a challenging task. Research on strategies that couples use to repair their marriages indicates that many couples lack effective strategies to turn the marriage around (Dindia & Baxter, 1987). The findings from my interviews on the marital disaffection process demonstrate that marital therapy must have different goals corresponding to each phase of the process of disaffection. An initial task of the clinician is to carefully assess both spouses for love toward the partner and commitment to the marriage to determine whether there is enough to build a stronger marriage. Then interventions can be chosen based on the phase of disaffection the spouses are in. Table 7.2 provides a summary of the interventions suggested for each phase of the disaffection process.

Suggestions for Future Research

In conclusion, I offer the following suggestions for future research in the area of marital disaffection. First, if we want to learn more about how love is maintained in a marriage, future studies need to also include in-depth interviews with a comparison group of spouses who are not disaffected. A group of nondisaffected spouses could be asked questions regarding early marital disillusionment, conflict resolution, coping with stressful events, and types of repair efforts. Another way to study how love is maintained or dies would be to conduct a longitudinal panel study in which the same spouses are followed over time. Perhaps this is the best way to see if love and affection actually decline, stay the same, or increase.

Second, we need to develop instruments (questionnaire, interview, observation tools) that can help us pinpoint where a person is in the disaffection process. The instrument would not only aid our understanding of the precursors of each phase of disaffection but would assist clinicians in determining exactly the phase the person is in and what interventions would have the best chance of working. Although the disaffection scale developed for the present study is adequate for determining the overall level of disaffection, it does not tell us what phase a person is in. For example, if a person receives a moderate score on disaffection, this does not necessarily mean he or she is in the middle phase.

Third, future studies could focus on the duality of the marital relationship, utilizing interviews with the partners of the disaffected

TABLE 7.2 Interventions during the Process of Marital Disaffection

Phases	Objectives	Interventions
Beginning	To teach relationship skills	Social skills training such as communication and conflict resolution (Garland, 1983; Gottman et al., 1976; Guerney, 1977; Jacobson & Margolin, 1979; L'Abate, 1977; Miller et al., 1976; Valle & Marinelli, 1975)
	To increase couple's awareness about marital contracts and resolve conflicting expectations	Work with marital contracts (Sager, 1981)
	To modify dysfunctional standards for marriage	Cognitive modification (Baucom & Epstein, 1990)
Middle	To increase the level of positive behavior exchange	"Caring Days" (Stuart, 1980), "Love Days" (Weiss et al., 1973), and behavioral contracts (Jacobson & Margolin, 1979)
	To recognize multiple factors responsible for marital problems	Cognitive restructuring and reattribution (Baucom, 1987; Baucom & Epstein, 1990; Beck, 1988; Epstein, 1983)
End	To address bitterness and anger	"Bitterness Protocol" (Guerin et al., 1987)
	To assist in making decision about marriage— repair or disengagement?	Diagnostic issues in decision making (Kressel, 1985); structured separation (Granvold, 1983; Rice & Rice, 1986)
	To facilitate disengagement, if it is desired, and postdivorce adjustment	Divorce mediation (Kressel et al., 1980; Steinberg, 1980); divorce recovery groups (Weiss, 1975)

spouses. These studies would provide additional information on discrepant views of the relationship. There are several different perspectives of a relationship—not only Olson's (1977) "insider" and "outsider" perspectives but two different "insider" perspectives (Duck & Sants, 1983). Knowing both "insider" perspectives could provide us with a clearer understanding of the problems in the relationship. Involving both partners in the study would provide information on the mutuality of disaffection; that is, to what extent both spouses are disaffected. One possibility to be explored is that both spouses are going through the process of disaffection, but one is "ahead" of the other. The apathy experienced by the spouse who is in the last phase may intensify the middle phase anger of his or her partner.

A fourth area for future study is research on the causes of disaffection. What societal factors impact the emotional bond of a couple? Indeed, greater anonymity, loose community ties, and economic pressures can place a couple under tremendous stress, which in turn produces greater demands on their relationship. Whereas stress may initially bring a couple closer together, over time it is likely to put undue strain on the relationship. Personality variables could also be explored as possible factors related to marital disaffection. Numerous researchers are currently studying different relationship styles based on early childhood attachments with parents (Bartholomew, 1990; Feeney & Noller, 1991; Hazen & Shaver, 1987; Senchak & Leonard, 1992). These researchers are interested in how mental models or schemas based on early stages of social development influence later adult relationships. Schwartz (1987) also links personality traits to spouses' ability to be intimate. Basically, the question is whether individuals with certain personality traits tend to be more susceptible to marital disaffection. Some disaffected spouses or their partners may have had difficulty maintaining love relationships in general.

Another area of research involves variations in the marital disaffection process due to time in each phase, phase sequences, and phase skipping. Are there some people who do not go through the phases in the sequence most typical of my sample? For example, some individuals may skip a phase or go through the phases several times, just repeating the process over again.

Clinical research in testing the effectiveness of interventions at particular stages of relationship breakdown is needed. Is the timing of certain interventions during the process of marital breakdown important? If, as Duck (1984) proposes, "there is a ripeness in the time for applying certain techniques," (p. 165) what interventions would be the most effective at what times? Based on my three-stage model of marital disaffection, I have suggested specific foci of therapy and interventions that may be applied. The effectiveness of the implementation of these suggested intervention techniques at each stage remains to be tested.

Finally, more work is needed to design and develop interventions to deal with unilateral disaffection or "polarized couples" (Crosby, 1989). Spouses may be in quite different places emotionally when they seek therapy. It is not uncommon to hear a spouse in therapy say, "I'm happy in the marriage; I don't see any problems," while the partner is talking about getting a divorce. Working with couples who differ widely in their levels of disaffection is a particular challenge for marital therapists. This discrepancy in the level of disaffection may be the primary reason for seeking therapy. If the spouses mutually agreed that they did not love each other, they would be likely to dissolve the marriage together rather than coming to therapy. Too often the disaffected spouse is pursuing counseling alone—before the partner is experiencing any marital dissatisfactions or any motivation for therapy. Only later does the partner become motivated to seek help. But at this point it is often too late as far as the disaffected spouse is concerned.

Questionnaire on Marital Relationships

This questionnaire is about your marital relationship. All answers are completely *confidential*. Please *do not write your name on the questionnaire*.

I. The following statements relate to feelings that spouses may have toward each other. Make an "X" in the column indicating how true the statement is in regards to the feelings you have toward your spouse: it is *very true, somewhat true, not very true,* or *not at all true.*

	Very True	Somewhat True	Not Very True	Not at All True
1. If I could never be with my spouse, I would feel miserable.				
2. I find it difficult to confide in my spouse about a number of things.				
3. I enjoy spending time alone with my spouse.				
4. I often feel lonely even though I am with my spouse.				
5. I miss my spouse when we're not together for a couple days.				
6. Most of the time I feel very close to my spouse.				

	Very True	Somewhat True	Not Very True	Not at All True
7. I seem to enjoy just being with my spouse.				
8. I look forward to seeing my spouse at the end of the day.				
9. My love for my spouse has increased more and more over time.				
10. I find myself withdrawing more and more from my spouse.				
11. When I have a personal problem, my spouse is the first person I turn to.				
12. Apathy and indifference best describe my feelings toward my spouse.				
13. I feel little, if any, desire to have sex with my spouse.				
14. My spouse has always been there when I needed him or her.				
15. I would prefer to spend less time with my spouse.				
16. I have more positive than negative thoughts about my partner.				
17. I have a lot of angry feelings toward my spouse.				
18. I am not as concerned about fulfilling my obligations and responsibilities in my marriage as I was in the past.				
19. I try to avoid spending time with my spouse.				

	Very True	Somewhat True	Not Very True	Not at All True
20. There are times when I do not feel a great deal of love and affection for my mate.				
21. I enjoy sharing my feelings with my spouse.				

II. The following is a list of things that *can contribute to problems in marriages.* For each, mark an "X" in the column which best indicates the extent to which it accounts for problems you have experienced in your marriage. *It is important that you answer every item.* If you think a particular item doesn't apply to you, answer "not at all."

	A Great Deal	A Fair Amount	Only a Little	Not at All
1. Stress with one or both partner's work or educational activities				
2. Moving to a new residence				
3. The death of a family member or close friend				
4. Financial problems				
5. The illness or disability of a spouse or family member				
6. Interference of in-laws				
7. Relationships with step-family members				
8. Birth of first child				
9. Birth of an additional child				
10. Child(ren) leaving home				
11. Retirement				
12. Unemployment				

	A Great Deal	A Fair Amount	Only a Little	Not at All
13. My spouse's emotional immaturity				
14. My spouse's lack of self-disclosure				
15. My spouse's selfishness				
16. My spouse's aggressiveness				
17. My spouse's passivity or withdrawal				
18. My spouse's depressed moods				
19. My spouse's substance abuse (alcohol or other drugs)				
20. My spouse's desire for more freedom or a new lifestyle				
21. My spouse's romantic involvement outside the marriage				
22. Other interests of my spouse outside the marriage				
23. My spouse's lack of motivation to make the marriage better				
24. My spouse's controlling behavior				
25. My own emotional immaturity				
26. My own lack of self-disclosure				
27. My own selfishness				
28. My own aggressiveness				
29. My own passivity or withdrawal				

Appendix A

	A Great Deal	A Fair Amount	Only a Little	Not at All
30. My own depressed moods				
31. My own substance abuse (alcohol or other drugs)				
32. My own desire for more freedom or a new lifestyle				
33. My romantic involvement outside the marriage				
34. Other interests of mine outside the marriage				
35. My own lack of motivation to make the marriage better				
36. My own controlling behavior				
37. Physical abuse between me and my spouse				
38. Verbal abuse between me and my spouse				
39. The way my spouse and I solve disagreements				
40. Being physically separated a great deal of time				
41. An unequal distribution of power				
42. Different personal values				
43. Inadequate communication				
44. Incompatibility in sexual relations				
45. Different expectations for marriages				
46. Conflict over educational aspirations and career or occupational goals				

III. Indicate to what extent each of the following items describes you. Circle 1 if you feel you are not at all like this; 10 if you think you are a lot like this; or circle any number in between.

	Not at all									A lot
1. Personally happy	1	2	3	4	5	6	7	8	9	10
2. Satisfied with life	1	2	3	4	5	6	7	8	9	10
3. Feeling tense	1	2	3	4	5	6	7	8	9	10
4. Feeling conflicted	1	2	3	4	5	6	7	8	9	10
5. Depressed	1	2	3	4	5	6	7	8	9	10
6. Optimistic	1	2	3	4	5	6	7	8	9	10
7. Self-confident	1	2	3	4	5	6	7	8	9	10
8. Successful	1	2	3	4	5	6	7	8	9	10
9. Socially active	1	2	3	4	5	6	7	8	9	10

IV. The following are general statements about married couples but not necessarily about your relationship. How much do you agree or disagree with each statement?

	Strongly agree									Strongly disagree
1. A member of a couple that has been together a long time should not accept a job he or she wants in a distant city if it means ending the relationship.	1	2	3	4	5	6	7	8	9	10
2. Couples should try to make their relationship last a lifetime.	1	2	3	4	5	6	7	8	9	10
3. Marriage is a lifetime relationship and should never be terminated except under extreme circumstances.	1	2	3	4	5	6	7	8	9	10

V. Please provide the following information about yourself. Remember that this and all other information will be kept strictly confidential.

1. Sex: _____   2. Age: _____
3. Length of marriage: _____
4. Have you been previously married?   Yes   No   (circle one)
5. Do you have any children from this marriage?   Yes   No
   If so, how many? _____   (circle one)
6. Do you have any children from a previous marriage?   Yes   No
   If so, how many? _____   (circle one)
7. What was the last year of school you completed? (circle number)
   1. Some grade school   5. Some college
   2. Finished grade school   6. Finished college
   3. Some high school   7. Attended graduate or
   4. Finished high school after   professional school
      college
8. Which figure comes closest to you and your spouse's combined yearly income: (circle number)
   1. $0–$4,999   7. $30,000–$39,999
   2. $5,000–$9,999   8. $40,000–$49,999
   3. $10,000–$14,999   9. $50,000–$59,999
   4. $15,000–$19,999   10. $60,000–$69,999
   5. $20,000–$24,999   11. $70,000–$79,999
   6. $25,000–$29,999   12. $80,000 and over
9. Have you been receiving counseling for marital problems during the last six months?   Yes   No   (circle one)

Thank you for taking time to complete the questionnaire. Don't forget to mail your postcard separately when you mail your questionnaire.

Interview Schedule

Each respondent will be asked to sign a statement of agreement to be interviewed. The introduction to the interview will also include statements that (a) the respondent understands that the interview is not part of any therapy, (b) the respondent understands that this information is for research purposes only, and (c) that his or her name or any other identification will not be used in connection with any statements regarding the interview.

I will be asking you questions regarding events, behaviors, and important turning points in your relationship with you spouse— from the time you first met your spouse to the present year. But first I would like to ask you some general questions regarding your relationship.

1. How long did you and your current spouse know each other before you were married?
2. Did you live together? If so, for how long?
3. How old were you when you married your current spouse? How old was your spouse?
4. How long have you been married to your present partner?
5. During the course of a marriage, certain events happen or behaviors sometimes take place which bother a spouse and which may produce some doubts about the partner. These may be major turning points regarding one's feelings about one's spouse. Take a moment to think about the first time you had

doubts about your spouse and the marriage. Tell me what happened.

5a. What year of your relationship did this occur?

5b. How long did this problem last?

6. Was there another major event which also produced some doubts about your partner?

    1. YES   2. NO
                     GO TO 7

    6a. Tell me what happened.

    6b. What year did this occur during your relationship?

    6c. How long did this problem last?

    (CONTINUE WITH REPEATING QUESTION 6 UNTIL NO OTHER EVENTS ARE REPORTED)

7. Now I would like to ask you more specific questions regarding each of these events. During the first event (REPEAT EVENT), tell me about the feelings you experienced regarding your spouse? How did you show your feelings? (PROBE—any other feelings respondent may have had)

    7a. What thoughts did you have regarding your (husband/wife) at this time (REPEAT EVENT)?

    (IF NECESSARY, GIVE DEFINITION AND EXAMPLE OF A THOUGHT—an idea or expectation, e.g., My marriage is not as happy as most people's)

    (PROBE—any other thoughts)

    7b. Tell me about any particular actions you took during this time (REPEAT EVENT)?

    (PROBE—any other actions)

    7c. What actions did your spouse take?

    7d. What did you think was the cause of this situation? What was responsible for the situation?

    7e. How did you cope with the situation?

8. REPEAT 7 FOR EACH SUBSEQUENT EVENT—During the second event (REPEAT EVENT), tell me about the feelings you experienced regarding your (wife/husband).

    8a. REPEAT 7a. (THOUGHTS).

8b. REPEAT 7b and 7c. (ACTIONS)
8c. REPEAT 7d. (CAUSE)
8d. REPEAT 7e. (COPING)

9. When did you first openly talk about marital dissatisfactions with your spouse?

10. What are your current feelings about your (husband/wife)?

11. What are your current thoughts about your (husband/wife)?

12. What actions are you taking relative to your marriage?

13. Are you currently satisfied with the relationship?
    1. YES   2. NO

    13a. What do you think   13b. What contributes *most* to
    accounts for the sat-   your dissatisfaction?
    isfaction you are
    currently experien-
    cing?

    GO TO 14   13c. What changes would need to
                             take place for you to feel bet-
                             ter about the marriage?

                             13d. Are any actions being taken
                             to make these changes?
                             1. YES   2. NO
                                           GO TO 14
                                           (RESIGNATION)

                             13e. What actions are being taken?
                             (REPAIR)

                             13f. Have these actions resulted in
                             any changes in your feelings
                             about your spouse?

14. Have you ever seriously considered the possibility of separation or divorce?
    1. YES   2. NO
    14a. When?   GO TO 15

15. Are any actions being taken to end the relationship?
    1. YES   2. NO
    (DISSOLUTION)

15a. What actions are being taken?   15b. What things are keeping you in the marriage?

16. Are you pursuing any alternatives to this marriage? (e.g., relationships with other people as a friend or lover)
    1. YES   2. NO
                    GO TO 17
    16a. What alternatives have you pursued?

17. Have you been involved in marriage counseling?
    1. YES   2. NO
                    GO TO 18
    17a. When was it initiated?
    17b. Was there a particular happening or event that caused counseling to be sought out?
    17c. Regarding the decision to seek marriage counseling, which statement best applies:
       (1) It was my idea to go a while ago but (his or hers) now.
       (2) It was (his or her) idea to go a while ago but mine now.
       (3) It was more my idea to go all along.
       (4) It was more my partner's idea to go all along.
       (5) We both equally wanted counseling.
       (6) It was neither spouse's idea to go.

18. How do you think your life would be different if you were not married?

References

Acitelli, L. K. (1992). Gender differences in relationship awareness and marital satisfaction among young married couples. *Personality and Social Psychology Bulletin, 18,* 102–110.

Albrecht, S. L., Bahr, H. M., & Goodman, K. L. (1983). *Divorce and remarriage: Problems, adaptations, and adjustments.* Westport, CT: Greenwood.

Andrews, B., & Brewin, C. R. (1990). Attributions of blame for marital violence: A study of antecedents and consequences. *Journal of Marriage and the Family, 52*(3), 757–767.

Aronson, E. (1970). Some antecedents of interpersonal attraction. In W. J. Arnold & D. Levine (Eds.), *Nebraska Symposium on Motivation, 1969.* Lincoln, NE: University of Nebraska Press.

Bardwick, J. M. (1979). *In transition.* New York: Holt, Rinehart & Winston.

Barnett, R. C., & Baruch, G. K. (1987). Mother's participation in child care: Patterns and consequences. In F. J. Crosby (Ed.), *Spouse, parent, worker: On gender and multiple roles* (pp. 63–73). New Haven, CT: Yale University Press.

Bartholomew, K. (1990). Avoidance of intimacy: An attachment perspective. *Journal of Social and Personal Relationships, 7*(2), 147–178.

Baucom, D. H. (1987). Attributions in distressed relations: How can we explain them? In D. Perlman & S. Duck (Eds.), *Intimate relationships: Development, dynamics, and deterioration* (pp. 177–206). Newbury Park, CA: Sage.

Baucom, D. H., & Epstein, N. (1990). *Cognitive-behavioral marital therapy.* New York: Brunner/Mazel.

Baxter, L. A. (1984). Trajectories of relationship disengagement. *Journal of Social and Personal Relationships, 1*(1), 29–48.

Beach, S. R. H. (1991). Social cognition and the relationship repair process: Toward better outcome in marital therapy. In G. J. O. Fletcher

& F. D. Fincham (Eds.), *Cognition in close relationships* (pp. 307–328). Hillsdale, NJ: Erlbaum.

Beck, A. T. (1988). *Love is never enough.* New York: Harper & Row.

Belenky, M. F., Clinchy, B. M., Goldberger, N. R., & Tarule, J. M. (1986). *Women's ways of knowing: The development of self, voice, and mind.* New York: Basic Books.

Benin, M. H., & Agostinelli, J. (1988). Husbands' and wives' satisfaction with the division of labor. *Journal of Marriage and the Family, 20,* 349–361.

Bepko, C., & Krestan, J. A. (1985). *Responsibility trap: A blueprint for treating the alcoholic family.* New York: Free Press.

Berardo, F. M. (1990). Trends and directions in family research. *Journal of Marriage and the Family, 52*(4), 809–817.

Berger, C. R., & Roloff, M. E. (1982). Thinking about friends and lovers: Social cognition and relational trajectories. In M. Roloff & C. Berger (Eds.), *Social cognition and communication* (pp. 151–192). Beverly Hills, CA: Sage.

Bernard, J. (1982). *The future of marriage.* New Haven, CT: Yale University Press.

Berscheid, E., & Campbell, B. (1981). The changing longevity of heterosexual close relationships: A commentary and forecast. In M. J. Lerner & C. S. Lerner (Eds.), *The justice motive in social behavior: Adapting to times of scarcity and change* (pp. 209–234). New York: Plenum Press.

Blood, R. O., & Wolfe, D. M. (1960). *Husbands and wives.* New York: Free Press.

Bloom, B. L., & Hodges, W. W. (1981). The predicament of the newly separated. *Community Mental Health Journal, 17,* 277–293.

Blumstein, P., & Schwartz, P. (1983). *American couples.* New York: Morrow.

Booth, A., Johnson, D. R., & Edwards, J. N. (1983). Measuring marital instability. *Journal of Marriage and the Family, 45*(2), 387–394.

Bradbury, T. N., & Fincham, F. D. (1990). Attributions in marriage: Review and critique. *Psychological Bulletin, 107*(1) 3–33.

Brown, P. (1976). *Psychological distress and personal growth among women coping with marital dissolution.* Unpublished doctoral dissertation, University of Michigan, Ann Arbor.

Brown, D. R., & Gary, L. E. (1985). Social support network differentials among married and nonmarried black females. *Psychology of Women Quarterly, 9,* 229–241.

Burgess, E. W., & Locke, H. J. (1945). *The family.* New York: American Book.

References

Buunk, B. (1987). Conditions that promote breakups as a consequence of extradyadic involvements. *Journal of Social and Clinical Psychology, 5*(3), 271–284.

Cahn, S., & Van Heusen, J. (1955). *Love and marriage*. Los Angeles, CA: Warner/Chappell Music. [Warner/Chappell Music, Inc. administers the rights on behalf of Cahn Music Co. and Baron Music Corp.]

Campbell, J. (1987). Cognitive dissonance. In R. J. Corsini (Ed.), *Concise encyclopedia of psychology* (pp. 208–209). New York: Wiley.

Campbell, A., Converse, D. E., & Rodgers, W. L. (1976). *The quality of American life*. New York: Sage.

Camper, P. M., Jacobson, N. S., Holtzworth-Munroe, A., & Schmaling, K. B. (1988). Causal attributions for interactional behaviors in married couples. *Cognitive Therapy and Research, 12*, 195–209.

Caplow, T., Bahr, H. M., Chadwick, H. R., & Williamson, M. H. (1982). *Middletown families: Fifty years of change and continuity* Minneapolis: University of Minnesota Press.

Carter, S., & Sokol, J. (1987). *Men who can't love: When a man's fear makes him run from commitment*. New York: M. Evans.

Chodorow, N. (1978). *The reproduction of mothering*. Berkeley: University of California Press.

Coverman, A., & Sheley, J. F. (1986). Change in men's housework and child-care time, 1965–1975. *Journal of Marriage and the Family, 48*, 413–422.

Cowan, R. S. (1987). Women's work, housework, and history: The historical roots of inequality in work-force participation. In N. Gerstel & H. E. Gross (Eds.), *Families and work* (pp. 164–177). Philadelphia: Temple University Press.

Crosby, J. F. (1985). *Illusion and disillusion: The self in love and marriage*. Belmont, CA: Wadsworth.

Crosby, J. F. (1989). *When one wants out and the other doesn't: Doing therapy with polarized couples*. New York: Brunner/Mazel.

Cuber, J. F., & Harroff, P. B. (1965). *Sex and the significant Americans*. New York: Appleton-Century.

Depner, C. E., & Ingersoll-Dayton, B. (1985). Conjugal social support: Patterns in later life. *Journal of Gerontology, 40*, 761–766.

Dindia, K., & Baxter, L. A. (1987). Strategies for maintaining and repairing marital relationships. *Journal of Social and Personal Relationships, 4*(2), 143–158.

Dizard, J. (1968). *Social change in the family*. University of Chicago: Community of Family Study Center.

Doherty, W. J., Lester, M. E., & Leigh, G. (1986). Marriage Encounter

References

weekends: Couples who win and couples who lose. *Journal of Marital and Family Therapy, 12*(1), 49–61.

Douglas, J. D., & Atwell, F. C. (1988). *Love, intimacy, and sex.* Newbury Park, CA: Sage.

Duck, S. (1981). Toward a research map for the study of relationship breakdown. In S. Duck & R. Gilmour (Eds.), *Personal relationships 3: Personal relationships in disorder* (pp. 1–29). London: Academic Press.

Duck, S. (1982). A topography of relationship disengagement and dissolution. In S. Duck (Ed.), *Personal relationships 4: Dissolving personal relationships* (pp. 1–30). London: Academic Press.

Duck, S. (1984). A perspective on the repair of personal relationships: Repair of what, when? In S. Duck (Ed.), *Personal relationships 5: Repairing personal relationships* (pp. 163–184). London: Academic Press.

Duck, S. (1988). *Relating to others.* Chicago, IL: The Dorsey Press.

Duck, S. W., & Sants, H. K. (1983). On the origin of the specious: Are personal relationships really interpersonal states? *Journal of Social and Clinical Psychology, 1,* 27–41.

Editor and Publisher Market Guide. (1988). New York: Editor and Publisher Co.

Eiser, J. R. (1983). Attribution theory and social cognition. In J. Jaspars, F. Fincham, & M. Hewstone (Eds.), *Attribution theory and research: Conceptual, developmental and social dimensions* (pp. 211–255). London: Academic Press.

Epstein, N. (1983). Cognitive therapy with couples. In A. Freeman (Ed.), *Cognitive therapy with couples and groups* (pp. 107–123). New York: Plenum Press.

Feeney, J. A., & Noller, P. (1991). Attachment style and verbal descriptions of romantic partners. *Journal of Social and Personal Relationships, 8*(2), 187–215.

Fincham, F. D., (1985). Attribution processes in distressed and nondistressed couples: 2. Responsibility for marital problems. *Journal of Abnormal Psychology, 94*(2), 183–190.

Fincham, F. D., & Beach, S. R. (1988). Attribution processes in distressed and nondistressed couples: 5. Real versus hypothetical events. *Cognitive Therapy and Research, 12,* 505–514.

Fincham, F. D., & O'Leary, K. D. (1983). Causal inferences for spouse behavior in maritally distressed and nondistressed couples. *Journal of Social and Clinical Psychology,* (1), 42–57.

Fletcher, G. (1983). The analysis of verbal explanation for marital separation: Implications for attribution theory. *Journal of Applied Social Psychology, 13*(3), 245–258.

References

Fletcher, G. J., Fincham, F. D., Cramer, L., & Heron, N. (1987). The role of attributions in the development of dating relationships. *Journal of Personality and Social Psychology, 53*, 481–489.

Gallagher, C. (1975). *The Marriage Encounter: As I have loved you*. Garden City, NY: Doubleday.

Garland, D. (1983). *Working with couples for marriage enrichment*. New York: Free Press.

Giblin, P., Sprenkle, D. H., & Sheehan, R. (1985). Enrichment outcome research: A meta-analysis of premarital, marital and family interventions. *Journal of Marital and Family Therapy, 11*(3), 257–271.

Gilligan, C. (1982). *In a different voice: Psychological theory and women's development*. Cambridge, MA: Harvard University Press.

Glick, P. C. (1989). The family life cycle and social change. *Family Relations, 38*(2), 123–129.

Glick, P. C., & Norton, A. J. (1971, May). Frequency, duration, and probability of marriage and divorce. *Journal of Marriage and the Family, 33*, 307–317.

Goode, W. J. (1956). *After divorce*. Glencoe, IL: Free Press.

Goode, W. J. (1966). Family disorganization. In R. K. Merton & R. A. Nisbet (Eds.), *Contemporary social problems* (pp. 479–552). New York: Harcourt Brace Jovanovich.

Gottman, J. M. (1979). *Marital interaction: Experimental investigations*. New York: Academic Press.

Gottman, J. M., & Krokoff, L. J. (1989). Marital interaction and satisfaction: A longitudinal view. *Journal of Consulting and Clinical Psychology, 57*(1), 47–52.

Gottman, J., Notarius, C., Gonso, J., & Markman, H. (1976). *A couple's guide to communication*. Champaign, IL: Research Press.

Gove, W. R. (1972). The relationship between sex roles, mental illness and marital status. *Social Forces, 51*, 34–44.

Gove, W. R., Hughes, M., & Style, C. B. (1983). Does marriage have positive effects on the well-being of the individual? *Journal of Health and Social Behavior, 24*, 122–131.

Gove, W. R., & Shin, H-C. (1989). The psychological well-being of divorced and widowed men and women: An empirical analysis. *Journal of Family Issues, 10*, 122–144.

Gove, W. R., Style, C. B., & Hughes, M. (1990). The effect of marriage on the well-being of adults: A theoretical analysis. *Journal of Family Issues, 11*(1), 4–35.

Granvold, D. K. (1983). Structured separation for marital treatment and decision-making. *Journal of Marital and Family Therapy, 9*(4), 403–412.

Graziano, W. G., & Musser, L. M. (1982). The joining and the parting of the ways. In S. W. Duck (Ed.), *Personal relationships 4: Dissolving personal relationships* (pp. 75–106). London: Academic Press.

Guerin, P. J., Fay, L. F., Burden, S. L., & Kautto, J. G. (1987). *The evaluation and treatment of marital conflict: A four-stage approach.* New York: Basic Books.

Guerney, B. G. (1977). *Relationship enhancement.* San Francisco: Jossey-Bass.

Gurin, G., Veroff, J., & Feld, S. C. (1960). *Americans view their mental health.* New York: Basic Books.

Hafner, R. J., & Miller, R. J. (1991). Essential hypertension: Hostility, psychiatric symptoms and marital stress in patients and spouses. *Psychotherapy and Psychosomatics, 56*, 204–211.

Hagestad, G. O., & Smyer, M. A. (1982). Dissolving long-term relationships: Patterns of divorcing in middle age. In S. Duck (Ed.), *Personal relationships 4: Dissolving personal relationships* (pp. 155–187). London: Academic Press.

Harvey, J. H., Wells, G. L., & Alvarez, M. D. (1978). Attribution in the context of conflict and separation in close relationships. In J. H. Harvey, W. Ickes, & R. F. Kidd (Eds.), *New directions in attribution research* (Vol. 2, pp. 235–260). Hillsdale, NJ: Erlbaum.

Hatfield, E., Traupmann, J., Sprecher, S., Utne, M., & Hay, J. (1985). Equity and intimate relations: Recent research. In W. Ickes (Ed.), *Compatible and incompatible relationships* (pp. 91–117). New York: Springer-Verlag.

Hazen, C., & Shaver, P. (1987). Romantic love conceptualized as an attachment process. *Journal of Personality and Social Psychology, 52*(3), 511–524.

Heaton, T. B., & Albrecht, S. L. (1991). Stable unhappy marriages. *Journal of Marriage and the Family, 53*(3), 747–758.

Heim, S. C., & Snyder, D. K. (1991). Predicting depression from marital distress and attributional processes. *Journal of Marital and Family Therapy, 17*(1), 67–72.

Hite, S. (1987). *Women and love: A cultural revolution in progress.* New York: Knopf.

Holtzworth-Munroe, A., & Jacobson, N. S. (1985). Causal attributions of married couples: When do they search for causes? What do they conclude when they do? *Journal of Personality and Social Psychology, 48*, 1398–1412.

Howe, G. W. (1987). Attributions of complex cause and the perception of marital conflict. *Journal of Personality and Social Psychology, 53*(6), 1119–1128.

Jack, D. C. (1991). *Silencing the self: Women and depression*. Cambridge, MA: Harvard University Press.

Jacobson, N. S., & Margolin, G. (1979). *Marital therapy: Strategies based on social learning and behavior exchange principles*. New York: Brunner/Mazel.

Jacobson, N. S., McDonald, D. W., Follette, W. C., & Berley, R. A. (1985). Attribution processes in distressed and nondistressed married couples. *Cognitive Therapy and Research, 9*(1), 35–50.

Johnson, M. P. (1982). Social and cognitive features of the dissolution of commitment to relationships. In S. Duck (Ed.), *Personal relationships 4: Dissolving personal relationships* (pp. 51–73). London: Academic Press.

Jordan, J. V. (1991). The meaning of mutuality. In J. V. Jordan, A. G. Kaplan, J. B. Miller, I. P. Stiver, & J. L. Surrey (Eds.), *Women's growth in connection* (pp. 81–96). New York: Guilford Press.

Kersten, K. K. (1988). Disaffection in marriage: Its perceived process and attributions. Unpublished doctoral dissertation, The University of Michigan, Ann Arbor.

Kersten, K. K., & Kersten, L. K. (1988). *Marriage and the family: Studying close relationships*. New York: Harper & Row.

Kessler, R. C., & Essex, M. (1982). Marital status and depression: The importance of coping resources. *Social Forces, 51*, 484–507.

Kiecolt-Glaser, J. K., Fisher, L. D., Ogrocki, P., Stout, J. C. et al. (1987). Marital quality, marital disruption, and immune function. *Psychosomatic Medicine, 49*(1), 13–34.

Kingsbury, N. M., & Minda, R. B. (1988). An analysis of three expected intimate relationship states: Commitment, maintenance, and termination. *Journal of Social and Personal Relationships, 5*, 405–422.

Kinsey, A. C., Pomeroy, W. B., Martin, C. E., & Gebhard, P. (1953). *Sexual behavior in the human female*. Philadelphia: Saunders.

Kitson, G. C. (1982, May). Attachment to the spouse in divorce: A scale and its application. *Journal of Marriage and the Family, 44*, 379–393.

Kitson, G. C. (with W. M. Holmes). (1992). *Portrait of divorce*. New York: Guilford Press.

Kitson, G. C., Babri, K. B., & Roach, M. J. (1985). Who divorces and why: A review. *Journal of Family Issues, 6*(3), 255–293.

Kitson, G. C., & Sussman, M. B. (1982). Marital complaints, demographic characteristics and symptoms of mental distress in divorce. *Journal of Marriage and the Family, 44*, 87–101.

Klein, D. M. (1993). *Marriage and family workbook*. Unpublished manuscript.

Kressel, K. (1985). *The process of divorce: How professionals and couples negotiate settlements.* New York: Basic Books.

Kressel, K., Jaffee, N., Tuchmon, B., Watson, C., & Deutsch, M. (1980). A typology of divorcing couples: Implications for mediation and the divorce process. *Family Process, 101*–116.

L'Abate, L. (1977). *Enrichment: Structured interventions with couples, families, and groups.* Washington, DC: University Press of America.

LaGaipa, J. J. (1982). Rules and rituals in disengaging from relationships. In S. W. Duck (Ed.), *Personal relationships 4: Dissolving personal relationships.* London: Academic Press.

Lederer, W. J., & Jackson, D. D. (1968). *The mirages of marriage.* New York: W. W. Norton.

Lee, G. R. (1988). Marital intimacy among older persons: The spouse as confidant. *Journal of Family Issues, 9,* 273–284.

Lee, L. (1984). Sequences in separation: A framework for investigating endings of the personal (romantic) relationship. *Journal of Social and Personal Relationships, 1*(1), 49–73.

Levenson, S. (1979). *You don't have to be in "Who's Who" to know what's what.* New York: Simon & Schuster.

Leventhal, G. S. (1980). What should be done with equity theory? New approaches to the study of fairness in social relationships. In K. J. Gergen, M. S. Greenberg, & R. Willis (Eds.), *Social exchange: Advances in theory and research* (pp. 27–55). New York: Plenum Press.

Levinger, G. (1976). A social psychological perspective on marital dissolution. *Journal of Social Issues, 32*(1), 21–47.

Levinger, G. (1979). A social exchange view on the dissolution of pair relationships. In R. L. Burgess & T. L. Huston (Eds.), *Social exchange in developing relationships* (pp. 169–193). New York: Academic Press.

Levinger, G. (1983). Development and change. In H. H. Kelley, E. Berscheid, A. Christensen, J. H. Harvey, T. L. Huston, G. Levinger, E. McClintock, L. A. Peplau, & D. R. Peterson (Eds.), *Close relationships* (pp. 315–359). New York: Freeman.

Lewis, R. A., & Spanier, G. B. (1979). Theorizing about the quality and stability of marriage. In W. R. Burr, R. Hill, F. I. Nye, & I. L. Reiss (Eds.), *Contemporary theories about the family* (Vol. 1, pp. 268–294). New York: Free Press.

Mace, D., & Mace, V. (1986). Marriage enrichment: Developing interpersonal potential. In P. W. Dail & R. H. Jewson (Eds.), *In praise of fifty years: The Groves Conference on the conservation of marriage and the family* (pp. 19–26). Lake Mills, IA: Graphic Publishing.

References

Mackey, R. A., & O'Brien, B. A. (1992). *The centrality of gender in understanding adaptability in seasoned marriages.* Unpublished manuscript, Boston College, Chestnut Hill.

Markman, H. J., Duncan, S. W., Storaasli, R. D., & Howes, P. W. (1987). The prediction of marital distress: A longitudinal investigation. In K. Hahlweg & M. J. Goldstein (Eds.), *Understanding major mental disorder: The contribution of family interaction research* (pp. 266–289). New York: Family Process Press.

Martin, T. C., & Bumpass, L. L. (1989). Recent trends in marital disruption. *Demography, 26,* 37–52.

McCall, G. J. (1982). Becoming unrelated: The management of bond dissolution. In S. W. Duck (Ed.), *Personal relationships 4: Dissolving personal relationships* (pp. 211–232). London: Academic Press.

McCubbin, H., & Patterson, J. (1982). *Family stress and coping.* Springfield, IL: Thomas.

Miller, R. (1982). *Marital dissolution: Paths to breakup.* Unpublished doctoral dissertation, University of Massachusetts, Amherst.

Miller, S., Nunnally, E. W., & Wackman, D. B. (1976). Minnesota couples communication program (MCCP): Premarital and marital groups. In D. Olson (Ed.), *Treating relationships* (pp. 21–39). Lake Mills, IA: Graphic Publishing Co.

Napier, A. (1988). *The fragile bond: In search of an equal and enduring marriage.* New York: Harper & Row.

Newman, H. (1981). Communication within ongoing intimate relationships: An attributional perspective. *Personality and Social Psychology Bulletin, 7*(1), 59–70.

Newman, H. M., & Langer, E. J. (1981). Post-divorce adaptation and the attribution of responsibility. *Sex Roles, 7*(3), 223–232.

Norton, A. J., & Glick, P. C. (1979). Marital instability in America: Past, present and future. In G. Levinger & O. C. Moles (Eds.), *Divorce and separation: Context, causes, and consequences* (pp. 6–19). New York: Basic Books.

Notarius, C. I., & Vanzetti, N. A. (1983). The marital agendas protocol. In E. E. Filsinger (Ed.), *Marriage and family assessment* (pp. 209–227). Beverly Hills, CA: Sage.

Nye, F. I., & Berardo, F. M. (1973). *The family: Its structure and interaction.* New York: Macmillan.

O'Connor, P., & Brown, G. W. (1984). Supportive relationships: Fact or fancy? *Journal of Social and Personal Relationships, 1*(2), 159–175.

Olson, D. H. (1977). Insiders' and outsiders' view of relationships: Research studies. In G. Levinger & H. L. Raush (Eds.), *Close relationships:*

Perspectives on the meaning of intimacy (pp. 115–135). Amherst, MA: University of Massachusetts Press.

Olson, D. H. (1983). How effective *is* marriage preparation? In D. R. Mace (Ed.), *Prevention in family services* (pp. 65–75). Beverly Hills, CA: Sage.

Orthner, D. K. (1990). The family in transition. In D. Blankenhorn, S. Bayme, & J. B. Elshtain (Eds.), *Rebuilding the nest: A new commitment to the American family* (pp. 93–118), Milwaukee, WI: Family Service America.

Paul, N. L., & Paul, B. (1986). *A marital puzzle: Transgenerational analysis in marriage counseling.* New York: Norton.

Pearlin, L. (1975). Sex roles and depression. In N. Datan (Ed.), *Life-span developmental psychology.* New York: Academic Press.

Peterson, D. R. (1983). Conflict. In H. H. Kelley, E. Berscheid, A. Christensen, J. H. Harvey, T. L. Huston, G. Levinger, E. McClintock, L. A. Peplau, & D. R. Peterson (Eds.), *Close relationships* (pp. 360–396). New York: Freeman.

Pineo, P. C. (1961). Disenchantment in the later years of marriage. *Marriage and Family Living, 23,* 3–11.

Ponzetti, J. J., & Cate, R. M. (1986). The developmental course of conflict in the marital dissolution process. *Journal of Divorce, 10,* 1–15.

Popenoe, D. (1990). Family decline in America. In D. Blankenhorn, S. Bayme, & J. B. Elshtain (Eds.), *Rebuilding the nest: A new commitment to the American family* (pp. 39–51). Milwaukee, WI: Family Service America.

Raush, H. L., Barry, W. A., Hertel, R. K., & Swain, M. A. (1974). *Communication, conflict, and marriage.* San Francisco: Jossey-Bass.

Reik, T. (1976). *Of love and lust.* New York: Pyramid Books.

Rice, D. G., & Rice, J. K. (1986). Separation and divorce therapy. In N. S. Jacobson & A. S. Gurman (Eds.), *Clinical handbook of marital therapy* (pp. 279–299). New York: Guilford Press.

Rollins, B. C., & Cannon, K. L. (1974). Marital satisfaction over the family life cycle: A reevaluation. *Journal of Marriage and the Family, 36*(2), 271–282.

Rubin, L. B. (1983). *Intimate strangers.* New York: Harper & Row.

Rubin, Z. (1973). *Liking and loving: An invitation to social psychology.* New York: Holt, Rinehart & Winston.

Rusbult, C. E. (1980). Commitment and satisfaction in romantic associations: A test of the investment model. *Journal of Experimental Social Psychology, 16,* 172–186.

Rusbult, C. E. (1987). Responses to dissatisfaction in close relationships: The exit-voice-loyalty-neglect model. In D. Perlman & S. Duck

(Eds.), *Intimate relationships: Development, dynamics, and deterioration* (pp. 209–238). Newbury Park, CA: Sage.

Ryan, J., & Hughes, M. (1989). *Marital status general life satisfaction: A cross-national comparison.* Unpublished manuscript, Virginia Polytechnic Institute and State University, Blacksburg.

Sabatelli, R. M. (1988). Exploring relationship satisfaction: A social exchange perspective on the interdependence between theory, research, and practice. *Family Relations, 37,* 217–222.

Sabatelli, R. M., & Cecil-Pigo, E. (1985). Relational interdependence and commitment in marriage. *Journal of Marriage and the Family, 47*(4): 931–945.

Sager, C. J. (1981). Couple therapy and marriage contracts. In A. S. Gurman & D. P. Kniskern (Eds.), *Handbook of family therapy* (pp. 85–130). New York: Brunner/Mazel.

Scanzoni, L. D., & Scanzoni, J. (1988). *Men, women, and change: A sociology of marriage and family.* New York: McGraw-Hill.

Schaefer, M. T., & Olson, D. H. (1981). Assessing intimacy: The PAIR inventory. *Journal of Marital and Family Therapy, 7,* 47–60.

Schwartz, M. (1987, May). *Desire and intimacy disorders.* Paper presented at the annual meeting of the American Association of Sex Educators, Counselors, and Therapists, New York.

Senchak, M., & Leonard, K. E. (1992). Attachment styles and marital adjustment among newlywed couples. *Journal of Social and Personal Relationships, 9*(1), 51–64.

Snyder, D. K., & Regts, J. M. (1982). Factor scales for assessing marital disharmony and disaffection. *Journal of Consulting and Clinical Psychology, 50,* 736–743.

Spanier, G. B., & Thompson, L. (1984). *Parting: The aftermath of separation and divorce.* Beverly Hills, CA: Sage.

Staines, G. L., & Libby, P. L. (1986). Men and women in role relationships. In R. D. Ashmore & F. K. DelBoca (Eds.), *The social psychology of female-male relations: A critical analysis of central concepts* (pp. 211–255). New York: Academic Press.

Steinberg, J. L. (1980). Towards an interdisciplinary commitment: A divorce lawyer proposes attorney-therapist marriages or, at the least, an affair. *Journal of Marital and Family Therapy, 6*(3), 259–268.

Stephen, T. (1987). Attribution and adjustment to relationship termination. *Journal of Social and Personal Relationships, 4*(1), 47–61.

Stuart, R. B. (1980). *Helping couples change.* New York: Guilford Press.

Swensen, C. H., Eskew, R. W., & Kohlhepp, K. A. (1981). Stage of family life cycle, ego development, and the marriage relationship. *Journal of Marriage and the Family, 43*(4), 841–853.

Swensen, C. H., & Moore, C. (1979). Marriages that endure. In E. Corfman (Ed.), *Families today: Strengthening the family* (Monograph No. 1). Rockville, MD: NIMH Science Monographs.

Swensen, C. H., & Trahaug, G. (1985). Commitment and the long-term marriage relationship. *Journal of Marriage and the Family, 47*(4), 939–945.

Szinovacz, M. E. (1984). Changing family roles and interactions. In B. B. Hess & M. B. Sussman (Eds.), *Women and the family: Two decades of change* (pp. 164–201). New York: Haworth Press.

Thibaut, J. W., & Kelley, H. H. (1959). *The social psychology of groups.* New York: Wiley.

Thoits, P. A. (1985). Social support and psychological well-being: Theoretical possibilities. In I. Sarason & B. Sarason (Eds.), *Social support: Theory, research and applications* (pp. 51–72). Dordrecht, The Netherlands: Martinus Nijhoff.

Thornes, B., & Collard, J. (1979). *Who divorces?* London: Routledge & Kegan Paul.

Toomim, M. K. (1972). Structured separation with counseling: A therapeutic approach for couples in conflict. *Family Process, 11,* 299–310.

Trost, J. E. (1986). What holds marriages together? *Acta Sociologica, 29*(4), 303–310.

Udry, J. R. (1966). Marital instability by race, sex, education, and occupation using 1960 census data. *American Journal of Sociology, 72,* 203–209.

U.S. Bureau of the Census. (1980). *1980 census of population and housing.* Washington, DC: Department of Commerce.

Valle, S. K., & Marinelli, R. P. (1975). Training in human relations skills as a preferred mode of treatment for married couples. *Journal of Marriage and Family Counseling, 1,* 359–365.

Vanfossen, B. E. (1986). Sex differences in depression: The role of spouse support. In S. E. Hobfoll (Ed.), *Stress, social support and women* (pp. 69–84). New York: Hemisphere.

Van Yperen, N. W., & Buunk, B. (1990). A longitudinal study of equity and satisfaction in intimate relationships. *European Journal of Social Psychology, 20,* 287–309.

Vaughan, D. (1986). *Uncoupling.* New York: Oxford University Press.

Veroff, J., Douvan, E., & Kulka, R. A. (1981). *The inner American.* New York: Basic Books.

Veroff, J., Kulka, R. A., & Douvan, E. (1981). *Mental health in America: Patterns of help-seeking from 1957–1976.* New York: Basic Books.

Walker, L. E. (1979). *The battered woman.* New York: Harper & Row.

Walster, E., Walster, G. W., & Berscheid, E. (1978). *Equity: Theory and research.* Boston: Allyn and Bacon.

References

Warner, R. L. (1986). Alternative strategies for measuring household division of labor: A comparison. *Journal of Family Issues,* 7, 179–195.

Weiss, R. L., Hops, H., & Patterson, G. R. (1973). A framework for conceptualizing marital conflict, technology, for altering it, some data for evaluating it. L. A. Hamerlynck, L. C. Handy, & E. J. Mash (Eds.), *Behavior change: Methodology, concepts, and practice.* Champaign, IL: Research Press.

Weiss, R. S. (1975). *Marital separation.* New York: Basic Books.

White, L. K. (1990). Determinants of divorce: A review of research in the eighties. *Journal of Marriage and the Family,* 52(4), 904–912.

Willits, F. K., & Crider, D. M. (1988). Health rating and life satisfaction in the later middle years. *Journal of Gerontology: Social Sciences,* 43(5), S172–176.

Witkin, S. L., Edelson, J. L., Rose, S. D., & Hall, J. A. (1983). Group training in marital communication: A comparative study. *Journal of Marriage and the Family,* 45, 661–669.

Yogev, S., & Brett, J. (1985). Perceptions of the division of housework and child care and marital satisfaction. *Journal of Marriage and the Family,* 47, 609–618.

Index

Affirmation, 121
Age, and marital stability, 12, 13, 24
Alienation, 3, 103, 121
Alternative attractions, 9–10, 18, 24, 56, 117
   awareness of, 114–116
Ambivalence, 21, 74, 90, 154–155
Anger, 14, 15, 20, 47–49, 65, 88, 89
   in beginning phase of disaffection, 90
   and blame attribution, 111
   replaced by apathy, 67, 68, 69, 159
   and unresolved conflicts, 104
Apathy, 6, 51, 67, 84, 89, 159
"As if" principle, 147–148
Association of Couples for Marital Enrichment, 141
Attachment, 121, 135
Attribution
   gender differences in, 105, 129, 130–131
   interpersonal, 129
   modifying, 149–152
   and phases of marital disaffection, 105–109, 149
   relationship, 129
   shifts in, 104–112, 127–131

testing validity of, 150–151
   theory, 126–127, 149
   types of, 104, 127
Avoidance, 87, 88, 104

B

Behavioral changes
   desired, 83–86
   positive, 148–149, 151, 158
"Bitter bank," 153
Bitterness, 152, 154, 158
   generational, 153
   protocol, 15, 152–154, 158
Blame; see Attribution, Self-blame

C

Caring, 121, 122, 135, 149
Children
   and divorce, 5, 56, 58, 73
   and marital stability, 12
Cognitive dissonance theory, 124–125, 135
Cognitive distortions, 150, 152
Cognitive focus, 52, 53, 56, 65, 88
Cognitive-Behavioral Marital Therapy (Baucom & Epstein), 147

Commitment, to marriage, 8–9, 10–12, 24, 73, 122
institutional vs. voluntary, 123–125, 135
shift in, 113
social vs. personal, 10–11
Communication, 7
breakdown of, 4, 100, 102
skills, 143
Communication Problem-Solving Workshops, 142
Compromise, 103
Conflict, in relationships, 14, 18, 83, 101–104, 116
in expectations, 145–146
withdrawal in, 102–103
Conflict resolution skills, 24, 104, 143, 144
Connection, need for, 37, 134
Controlling behavior, 93–100, 107
and decision-making process, 94, 98
and traditional gender roles, 98, 99–100
Coping strategies, 41–44, 86–88
denial as, 42, 87, 88
gender differences in, 87–88
self-punitive, 43–44
withdrawal as, 63, 79
Counseling; *see* Marital therapy
Couple's Communication Program, 142
Courtship, 33–34, 52, 54

D

Defensive behaviors, 82–83
Denial, 40, 42, 45, 80, 81–82, 87, 88
of self, 112–114
Depression, 121, 122, 134

Disaffection scale, 8, 22, 24–25n1, 157
Disenchantment; *see* Disillusionment
Disillusionment, 2, 20, 29, 32–35, 44, 45, 65
and changing perceptions, 33–34, 44–45, 145
short-term, 17
Distortion, need-related, 34, 52
Divorce, 2, 5–6, 10, 75
accounting for, 86
barriers to, 12, 24, 56–59, 73, 75
and behavioral changes, 83
emotional, 10
most common period for, 141
no-fault, 4
rate, in United States, 5, 8
reasons for, 4, 9
Divorce recovery programs, 156, 158
Dysfunctional relationship standards, 146–147, 158

E

Empathy, 95–96; *see also* Mutuality
Empty shell marriage, 59–60
Evaluation and Treatment of Marital Conflict, The (Guerin et al.), 152
Exchange theory, 55
Extradyadic attributions, 104, 105–107, 126, 127, 128, 149

F

Fantasy
loss of, 69–70
as solution, 152
Figure–ground hypothesis, 53

G

Growth in Marriage for
    Newlyweds, 141
Guilt, 69, 85, 88, 108

H

Happiness, marital, 113–114, 125,
    135
Household work, division of,
    133–134
Hurt, feelings of, 20, 49–52, 56,
    65, 88, 89
    and lack of mutuality, 96–97
    protection against, 53, 63, 79
    and unresolved conflicts, 104

I

Illusionary intimacy, 34, 145
Indifference; *see* Apathy
Interactive attribution, 104, 110,
    111, 127, 128–130, 135,
    136
Intermarital taboo, 43, 142–143
Intimacy
    emotional, 100–101, 116, 120,
        122, 132, 133, 135
    illusionary, 34, 145
    and personality traits, 159
Intimidation, 101; *see also* Control-
    ling behavior
Investment, in relationship, 9

L

Loneliness, 70, 88, 101, 116

M

Marital contracts, conflicting,
    145–146, 158
Marital disaffection, 6–24, 45
    alternatives to, 10, 18, 24, 56,
        114–116
    barriers to, 9, 18
    causes of, 93–117
    and family, 107, 147, 153
    future research on, 157, 159–
        160
    and gender, 131–135
    pathways to, 18
    and personality traits, 159
    phases of, 89–90, 116, 144,
        159–160
    and psychological well-being,
        120–138, 139
    questionnaire on, 21, 22, 26n2
    and reactions of nondisaffected
        partner, 38–41, 64, 80–85
    recovery from, 13–15
    research on, 17–23, 26–27n3–4
    sharing, 70–71
    spousal differences in, 14–17,
        24, 25–26n2
    theoretical model of, 19–21, 23,
        24, 90
    unilateral, 15–17, 24, 81, 160
    variations in, 8–17
Marital dissolution, 7; *see also*
    Divorce
    actions, 74–75
    decisions about, 71–74, 154–155
    final phase of, 76–88
    initiating, 85
    therapy in, 155–156
Marital doubts, 29–31, 41, 42; *see
    also* Turning point events
Marital expectations, 145–147
Marital Satisfaction Inventory, 7

Marital status, 2
and immune function, 5
and psychological well-being,
120, 131, 134–135
Marital therapy, 6, 13, 76–78, 88,
89, 139–160
for end phase, 152–156
hidden agendas in, 156
motivation for, 76, 78, 83, 160
as prevention, 140–147
and revival, 147–152
timing of, 160
Marriage
affective variables in, 4
changed criteria for, 2, 4
expectations of, 2–3, 32, 145–
147, 153
interpersonal processes in, 11, 94
love in, 3–4, 10, 23
1950s–1970s, 1
and psychological well-being,
120
sex role norms in, 97, 98–100
statistics on, 2
in the United States, 3–4
Marriage Encounter, 142
Marriage enrichment programs,
141–142
Mastery, sense of, 121, 135
Modifying attributions for
marital events, 149–152
Mutuality, 93–94, 95–96, 99–100,
116
and self-concept, 96–97
in woman-to-woman relationships, 99

N

Negative behavior, focus on, 52–
54, 65, 88, 90, 110

Negative reciprocity, 83, 103, 150
Neglect response, 12–13
Nonmarital cohabitation, 2

O

*One Wants Out and the Other
Doesn't* (Crosby), 16

P

Partner attributions, 104, 107–110,
111–112, 117, 127–130,
135, 136
and bitterness, 153
and hopelessness, 110
and marital therapy, 149–150,
151–152
positive, 151–152
Passive-aggressive behavior, 49
Passive–congenial marriage, 6
Personal Assessment of Intimacy
of Relationships, 24*n*1
Pity, for spouse, 69, 88, 110
Positive exchanges, 148–149
Power, 97, 99; *see also* Controlling
behavior, Mutuality
Premarital programs, 142
Problem-solving behavior, 60, 65,
76, 88, 89
failed, 102
resistance to, 83
Psychoeducational couples programs, 142
Psychotherapy, 143

Q

Questionnaire on Marital Rela-

tionships, 119, 123, 161–
166
sample responding, 119–120,
137–138

R

Reciprocal negativity; *see* Negative
reciprocity
Relational efficacy, 14
Relational thinking, 130, 137
Relationship Enhancement, 142
Responsibility, and marital prob-
lems, 36–38, 45, 78–79
attribution of; *see* Attribution
Reward–cost ratio, 54–56, 59–60,
65, 79, 89
Role theory, 122
Romantic love, 3, 4, 100, 143

S

Self-attribution; *see* Self-blame
Self-blame, 36–37, 107, 108, 109,
127, 149
Self-esteem, 61, 62, 96, 122, 126
and intimacy, 120, 122, 133
Self-fulfillment movement, 2
Separation, 63, 85, 155, 158
contract, 155
Sex, 4
extramarital, 4, 128

and withdrawal, 63, 101
Social contact, and marital stabil-
ity, 12
Social network, 71, 86, 88
Social skills training, 143–145,
158
Social validation, 70–71, 78, 87
Substance abuse, 41, 57, 60–61
and loss of intimacy, 101
Suicide, 43, 68

T

Teaching interpersonal skills, 143–
145
Tunnel vision, 150
Turning point events, 30–31, 94

V

Victim behavior, 153
Vigilance, 52, 65

W

Withdrawal, 38, 39, 62–63, 65, 89,
102–103
physical, 65, 79, 89
sexual, 63, 101